MEDICAL EXAMINATION REVIEW BOOK

E. C. F. M. G. EXAMINATION REVIEW

PART TWO

Fourth Edition

4 COMPLETE EXAMINATIONS
1,440 MULTIPLE CHOICE QUESTIONS
AND COMPLETELY REFERENCED
ANSWERS

Edited by

WARNER F. BOWERS, M.D., M.Sc., Ph.D.

MARVIN I. GOTTLIEB, M.D., Ph.D.

GERARD HELLMAN, M.D.

RICHARD LUMIERE, M.D.

GERALD WEINSTEIN, M.D.

NATHANIEL WISCH, M.D.

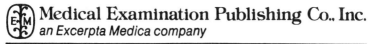 Medical Examination Publishing Co., Inc.
an Excerpta Medica company

969 Stewart Avenue   •   Garden City, New York 11530

MEDICAL EXAMINATION
REVIEW BOOK

E. C. F. M. G. EXAMINATION
REVIEW

PART TWO

FOURTH EDITION

TABLE OF CONTENTS

EDITORS

Warner F. Bowers, M.D., M.Sc., Ph.D., FACS
Formerly, *Professor of Clinical Surgery* and *Director,*
Graduate School of Medical Sciences
New York Medical College
New York, New York

with the assistance of

Gerald Weinstein, M.D.
Department of Surgery
Lenox Hill Hospital
New York, New York

Marvin I. Gottlieb, M.D., Ph.D., FAAP
Professor of Pediatrics
Director, Leigh Buring Memorial Clinic for Exceptional
   Children
University of Tennessee Center for the Health Sciences
Memphis, Tennessee

Richard M. Lumiere, M.D.
Attending Gynecologist and Obstetrician
Lenox Hill Hospital
   and
Attending Gynecologist
New York Fertility Research Foundation
New York, New York

Nathaniel Wisch, M.D.
Assistant Clinical Professor of Medicine
Mount Sinai School of Medicine of
   The City University of New York
New York, New York

with the assistance of

Gerard Hellman, M.D.
Fellow in Hematology, Department of Medicine
Mount Sinai Medical Center
New York, New York

INTRODUCTION

This book is being published as a supplement to Part One.

There are no shortcuts in the process of obtaining a medical education. Only a concerted effort, extensive study and review, and a willingness to learn can prepare an applicant for a comprehensive examination. Therefore, the authors of this text strongly advise the reader to first master the materials from accepted textbooks of medicine before attempting to test their powers of recall which are challenged by a "question and answer" review. After preparing for an examination by the proper time-tested method of study, this text becomes a valuable adjunct in your final preparation for a comprehensive test.

What then are the aims of the "question and answer" review? Several valuable purposes are achieved by such a test, which will better prepare the applicant for the *Educational Council for Foreign Medical Graduates Qualification Examination*. The authors have compiled fourteen-hundred-and-forty original, thought-provoking questions in the various fields encompassed by the qualification examination: Medicine, Pediatrics, Surgery, Obstetrics and Gynecology. The questions are designed to expose those areas of weakness which exist in your preparation. It is the intent of the authors to help you approach such areas of weakness by a mature process of learning. Consequently, this book has been designed not only to provide the reader with the correct answer, but, of greater value, each question is fully referenced from an accepted and standard medical textbook. To simply look up the correct answer to a given question is an ineffectual method of studying; rather, you are encouraged to return to the textbook to fortify your reservoir of knowledge by reading the section from which the question was derived. By utilizing this approach to the "question and answer" review, a question incorrectly answered becomes a stimulus for further study. Unlike other texts of this nature, the emphasis is on *additional* review of material from textbooks – a method of build a more substantial foundation for your store of medical knowledge.

Many fine textbooks are available to the physician for purposes of learning and review. The value of thoroughly reading your textbooks cannot be overemphasized. For the purposes of this examination review book, the authors have selected reference sources which number among the most widely used textbooks in the United States today. A list of these references is given in the back of this book.

Another objective of this review book is to familiarize the applicant with the language and mechanics of the E.C.F.M.G. Examination. Many of the needless fears and apprehensions about taking and preparing for an examination are eliminated when the applicant is confident that he has a complete understanding of the nature and meaning of the question. Undoubtedly, this may be an extremely important factor in determining your ability to successfully complete the examination. This book, by virtue of the large number of questions and the originality of the questions, provides you with an opportunity to familiarize yourself with the language and format of the objective type examination utilized by the *Educational Council for Foreign Medical Graduates*. This text can be regarded as a practice session which will enable you to feel at ease with the objective type examination. After mastering the design and directions of such an examination you will be able to more efficiently utilize your time in recalling medical information, rather than attempting to understand the meaning of the question itself. Learning the mechanics of a question prior to actually taking the qualification examination will give you more confidence in your ability to demonstrate the fund of medical knowledge which you have accumulated.

The authors once again wish to stress the concept that this review is not a substitute for a thorough preparation from accepted medical textbooks, nor is it designed to teach you all that is to be learned about the various medical fields tested for in the qualification examination. However, with a thorough comprehension of medical information, a working knowledge of the mechanics of the text and an understanding of the language of the examination you will be better equipped to pass the *Educational Council for Foreign Medical Graduates Examination*.

This book has been divided into four complete examinations similar to the E.C.F.M.G. examination. Each examination has been designed to cover all areas of study with all of the multiple-choice questions utilized on the actual examination.

If, after you have completed this volume, you feel that you would like to devote more time to certain subjects, please refer to some of our Medical Examination and Basic Science Review Books listed in the back of this book.

FIRST EXAMINATION

For each of the following multiple choice questions, select the one most appropriate answer:

1. Which one of the following cord blood tests would be of least value in evaluating a newborn with erythroblastosis:
   A. Direct Coomb's test
   B. Hemoglobin and hematocrit
   C. Reticulocyte and nucleated red cell count
   D. Indirect and total bilirubin levels
   E. Serum IgM levels   Ref. 10 - p. 64

2. Which one of the following findings is usually not commonly found in cor pulmonale with heart failure?
   A. Low pulmonary artery pressure
   B. High right ventricular end-diastolic pressure
   C. Right ventricular protodiastolic gallop
   D. Right ventricular hypertrophy
   E. Systemic venous congestion   Ref. 1 - p. 1332

3. Calculate the Apgar score from the following description: infant appears blue and pale, pulse rate 70/min., no response to stimulation of sole of foot by a brisk slap, limp muscle tone and slow-irregular respirations:
   A. 0   D. 7
   B. 2   E. 8
   C. 4   Ref. 10 - p. 71

4. After careful removal of all apparently involved tissue in cases of tuberculous tenosynovitis, it is good to give a course of anti-tuberculosis drug therapy because:
   A. Even the most careful dissection is apt to leave some diseased tissue
   B. Recurrence rate is high
   C. There may be other tuberculous foci
   D. All are correct
   E. Only A and B are true   Ref. 6 - p. 1850

5. Which of the following skin tests if positive usually suggests sarcoidosis?
   A. Tuberculin skin test   D. Bentonite flocculation test
   B. Kveim test   E. None of the above
   C. Skin test with Frei antigen   Ref. 1 - p. 1059

6. Gastric cancer occurs with increased frequency in patients of blood group:
   A. A   D. B
   B. O   E. Kell
   C. Rh-   Ref. 2 - p. 1293

11

12/First Examination

C   7. The most common location of carcinoma of the esophagus is:
       A. Upper third   D. Esophagogastric junction
       B. Middle third   E. Hiatus hernia
       C. Lower third   Ref. 2 - p. 1291

D   8. All of the following are characteristic of the infant that is small
        for gestational age, __except__:
       A. Hypoglycemia
       B. Congenital anomalies
       C. Anemia
       D. Chronic intrauterine infection
       E. Fetal distress leading to CNS depression
                                        Ref. 10 - p. 114

D   9. Hypocaloric dwarfism may result from:
       A. Intestinal malabsorption
       B. Chronic renal insufficiency
       C. Errors in preparing infant formulas
       D. All of the above
       E. None of the above   Ref. 10 - p. 170

D   10. A striking increase in the concentration of sodium and chloride
        in sweat is characteristic of:
       A. Adrenal cortical hyperplasia D. Cystic fibrosis of the pan-
       B. Primary aldosteronism   creas
       C. Villous adenoma of the rectum E. Chronic cholecystitis
                                        Ref. 2 - p. 1253

B   11. Cephalosporins may be used successfully against:
       A. Most pseudomonas infections   D. Shigella
       B. Enterobacter   E. None of the above
       C. Klebsiella   Ref. 1 - p. 745

E   12. The most common presenting manifestation of hypothyroidism
        in childhood is:
       A. Recurrent seizures   D. Laryngospasm
       B. Stiffness of hands   E. Cataracts
       C. Carpopedal spasm   Ref. 10 - p. 212

D   13. Concerning pica:
       A. In most cases craving is related to a dietary deficiency
       B. Usually causes severe gastrointestinal disturbances
       C. Usually treated by restraint
       D. All of the above
       E. None of the above   Ref. 10 - p. 271

D   14. Compounds inducing hemolysis of G6PD deficient erythrocytes:
       A. Acetanilid   D. All of the above
       B. Nitrofurantoin   E. None of the above
       C. Sulfanilamide   Ref. 10 - p. 395

C

15. The most common type of congenital tracheo-esophageal fistula is:
A. Proximal esophagus to trachea and atresia of distal esophagus
B. "H"-type
C. Atresia of proximal esophagus and distal tracheo-esophageal fistula
D. Both proximal and distal tracheo-esophageal fistulas
E. None of the above   Ref. 4 - p. 1171

B

16. Blood in the stool in the pediatric age group is almost never the result of:
A. Meckel's diverticulum   D. Anal fissure
B. Carcinoma   E. Juvenile polyps
C. Intussusception   Ref. 4 - p. 1186

E

17. The lesion often simulating primary bone tumor is:
A. Eosinophilic granuloma   D. Hyperparathyroidism
B. Fibrous dysplasia of bone E. All of the above
C. Paget's disease   Ref. 6 - p. 1771

B

18. The usual cause of chronic breast abscess is:
A. Tuberculosis   D. Actinomycosis
B. Staph aureus   E. Sarcoidosis
C. Inflammatory carcinoma   Ref. 4 - p. 577

B

19. The most common site for carcinoma of the breast is:
A. Nipple   D. Lower outer quadrant
B. Upper outer quadrant   E. Lower inner quadrant
C. Upper inner quadrant   Ref. 4 - p. 593

A

20. Decreased cardiac output is not evidenced by:
A. Pain   D. Edema
B. Dyspnea   E. Cyanosis
C. Fatigue   Ref. 6 - p. 749

B

21. Mucocele of the appendix is a(n):
A. Low grade malignancy   D. Allergic condition
B. Retention cyst   E. Low grade infection
C. Benign tumor   Ref. 6 - p. 1176

E

22. Implantation bleeding is called:
A. Hassin's sign   D. Hall's sign
B. Hoffman's sign   E. Hahn's sign
C. Hartman's sign   Ref. 7 - pp. 504-505

D

23. Prophylactic INH therapy may be indicated in:
A. Recent "converters" from a negative to a positive tuberculin skin test in whom there is no clinical or radiographic evidence of infection
B. Young children who react to tuberculin skin test
C. Household contacts of an open case of tuberculosis
D. All of the above
E. None of the above   Ref. 1 - p. 870

L

24. The disorder associated with the highest frequency of coarctation
of the aorta is:
   A. Turner's syndrome   D. "Rubella syndrome"
   B. Cretinism   E. Idiopathic infantile hyper-
   C. Down's syndrome   calcemia
                                    Ref. 1 - p. 578

A

25. Rocky Mountain spotted fever may be prevented in certain in-
stances by careful and rapid removal of:
   A. Ticks   D. Flies
   B. Mites   E. Fleas
   C. Lice   Ref. 2 - p. 257

B

26. Major trauma or sepsis may increase nutritional requirements:
   A. Not at all   D. 500-600%
   B. 200-300%   E. 800-900%
   C. 300-400%   Ref. 4 - p. 151

B

27. Which one of the following would be least expected in a child with
cystic fibrosis of the pancreas:
   A. Abnormal stool and eating patterns, often from birth
   B. Markedly decreased appetites in infants
   C. Respiratory infections and poor weight gain
   D. Cough
   E. Episodes of congestive failure later in childhood
                                    Ref. 10 - pp. 418-420

E

28. Which of the following are changes occurring normally in preg-
nancy with respect to renal function:
   A. Increased GFR   D. None
   B. Increased renal plasma flow E. All
   C. Bilateral ureteral dilatation Ref. 7 - p. 263

C

29. A retrodisplaced uterus:
   A. Has little effect on pregnancy
   B. Is a frequent cause of backache
   C. Produces few symtpoms in menopausal women
   D. Is a common cause of infertility
   E. Is most frequently congenital in nature
                                    Ref. 8 - p. 306

30. Migratory thrombophlebitis resistant to anticoagulants is suggestive of:

B

   A. Carcinoma of the pancreas D. Acute cholecystitis
   B. Biliary cirrhosis   E. Perforated ulcer
   C. Mallory-Weiss syndrome   Ref. 2 - p. 1254

D

31. Common sequelae of vaginal hysterectomy with anterior and
posterior colporrhaphy include:
   A. Urinary retention   D. All
   B. Acute cystitis   E. None
   C. Chronic cystitis   Ref. 8 - p. 115

D   32. Approximately ____ % of monozygotic twins of schizophrenic patients will show evidence of schizophrenia.
    A. .1   D. 50
    B. 1   E. 100
    C. 10   Ref. 2 - p. 565

⧫ E 33. D-Tubocurarine (curare) may be reversed by:
    A. Atropine   D. Gallamine
    B. Succinylcholine   E. Neostigmine
    C. Scopolamine   Ref. 4 - p. 205

    34. Which one of the following statements regarding melioidosis is not true?
    A. The disease may be asymptomatic
    B. Upper lobes of the lungs are almost never involved
    C. Cavitation of the pulmonary lesions frequently occurs
    D. Tetracycline is usually effective in the treatment of the disease
    E. Nodular skin lesions may be present
                                  Ref. 1 - p. 828

C   35. The most frequently encountered complaint with serous otitis media:
    A. Headache (temporal area)   D. "Popping" noise in the ear
    B. Sensation of fluid in the ear   E. Watery discharge from the
    C. Impairment of hearing   ear
                                  Ref. 10 - p. 462

B   36. If several ribs are fractured anteriorly and posteriorly, which is false?
    A. Tracheostomy usually is advisable
    B. Strapping of the chest is best
    C. Assisted positive pressure respiration may be needed
    D. Towel clip traction on the fracture segment is used
    E. Novocain intercostal nerve block relieves respiratory pain
                                  Ref. 6 - p. 604

D   37. Which one of the following antibiotics is penicillinase resistant?
    A. Aqueous penicillin   D. Methicillin
    B. Procaine penicillin   E. None of the above
    C. Paromomycin   Ref. 1 - p. 745

A   38. After any laparotomy in which small bowel is handled, there is a several day period of:
    A. Paralytic ileus   D. Fluid exudation
    B. Mechanical ileus   E. Calcium fixation
    C. Serositis   Ref. 6 - p. 990

A 39. A class V pap smear:
   A. Patient has definite malignant cells
   B. Patient has an invasive cancer
   C. Patient has a pre-invasive cancer
   D. Has a 10% error rate
   E. None of the above   Ref. 8 - p. 792

C 40. A characteristic clinical manifestation of schizophrenia is:
   A. Confusion   D. Visual hallucinations
   B. Anxiety   E. None of the above
   C. Auditory hallucinations   Ref. 2 - p. 564

D 41. Mania may be treated with:
   A. Lithium   D. All of the above
   B. Chlorpromazine   E. None of the above
   C. Haloperidol   Ref. 2 - p. 569

A 42. Which one of the following is to be avoided in the management of
   atopic eczema:
   A. Wet dressings
   B. Ointments containing corticosteroids
   C. Systemic treatment with antihistamines
   D. Barbiturates and sedative drugs
   E. A salve with 1 to 5 per cent tar   Ref. 10 - p. 474

B 43. The zone of fibrinoid degeneration where the trophoblast meets
   the decidua is called:
   A. Mayer's Membrane   D. Folds of Hoboken
   B. Nitabuch's Layer   E. Decidua Parietalis
   C. Chorionic Basement Membrane   Ref. 7 - p. 154

A 44. Following delivery human chorionic gonadotropin disappears
   from the serum within:
   A. 48 hours   D. Six weeks
   B. One week   E. Unknown
   C. Two weeks   Ref. 9 - p. 507

B 45. Which one of the following statements regarding poliomyelitis
   is true?
   A. It is usually not spread by the fecal-oral route
   B. Tonsillectomy is associated with an increase in the incidence
      of bulbar involvement
   C. The spinal fluid sugar is usually decreased
   D. Signs of upper motor neuron involvement are consistently
      present
   E. Vaccine is ineffective in prophylaxis
                           Ref. 1 - p. 951

D 46. Negri bodies are found in patients infected with:
   A. Measles   D. Rabies
   B. Yellow fever   E. Viral hepatitis
   C. Toxoplasmosis   Ref. 1 - p. 957

47. In regard to spinal cord tumors, which statement is true?
    A. Metastatic tumors usually are intradural
    B. About 2/3 of intradural tumors are benign and extramedullary
    C. Most cord tumors arise from neural elements
    D. Intramedullary tumors shell-out readily
    E. Intramedullary tumors rarely are cystic
    Ref. 6 - p. 1649

48. A retroverted uterus may be:
    A. Congenital
    B. Associated with endometriosis
    C. Associated with chronic pelvic infection
    D. All
    E. None
    Ref. 8 - p. 305

49. All of the following are regarded as major manifestations of rheumatic fever (Jones' criteria), except for:
    A. Carditis   D. Subcutaneous nodules
    B. Prolonged P-R interval   E. Chorea
    C. Erythema marginatum   Ref. 10 - p. 500

50. Leucine aminopeptidase is elevated with obstruction of the:
    A. Nasolacrimal duct   D. External auditory canal
    B. Common bile duct   E. Spermatic vein
    C. Ureter   Ref. 2 - p. 1317

51. The primary differential diagnosis of acute arthritis should include:
    A. Rheumatic fever   D. All of the above
    B. Serum sickness   E. None of the above
    C. Systemic lupus erythematosus   Ref. 10 - p. 514

52. How often does kernicterus occur if the bilirubin of the newborn rises to 20-30 mg%?
    A. 10%   D. 40%
    B. 20%   E. 50%
    C. 30%   Ref. 7 - p. 1047

53. The substance responsible for the gastrointestinal disturbances of carcinoid syndrome is:
    A. Cystokinen   D. Serotonin
    B. Rennin   E. Thyrocalcitonin
    C. Secretin   Ref. 6 - p. 1098

54. A seriously damaged myocardium may be thrown into ventricular fibrillation or cardiac arrest by:
    A. Endotracheal suctioning   D. Vagal stimulation
    B. Insertion of nasogastric tube   E. Any of the above
    C. Vomiting   Ref. 6 - p. 760

E 55. The most subtle sign of limited cardiac output is:
- A. Dyspnea
- B. Pink frothy sputum
- C. Pain
- D. Edema
- E. Fatigue

Ref. 6 - p. 750

56. Which one of the following statements is not true of schizophrenia?

C
- A. Hallucinations may be present
- B. Delusions may be present
- C. The patient is usually unconscious during an acute episode
- D. Symptoms begin most commonly during adolescence and early adulthood
- E. The phenothiazine group of drugs is often useful in therapy

Ref. 2 - p. 564

E 57. Mammography is particularly useful in which instance?
- A. Mass screening examinations
- B. Followup of contralateral breast after radical mastectomy
- C. Examination of indeterminate mass, especially among multiple cysts
- D. The large, fatty breast, difficult to palpate
- E. All of the above

Ref. 6 - p. 532

58. The best immediate treatment of frostbite is:

A
- A. Rewarming in water at 110-112 degrees F
- B. Packing the part in snow for slow thawing
- C. Brisk massage of the part to restore circulation
- D. Immediate excision of frozen tissue
- E. Immediate sympathetic nerve block

Ref. 6 - p. 905

C 59. A child with unexplained ataxia should be suspected of intoxica-
tion with:
- A. Lead
- B. Muscarine
- C. Salicylates
- D. Nitrates
- E. Cocaine

Ref. 10 - p. 533

60. Measures useful in the management of a case of tetanus may
include:

E
- A. Human tetanus immune globulin
- B. Penicillin
- C. Sedatives
- D. Tracheostomy
- E. All of the above

Ref. 1 - pp. 845-848

61. Best indication for closed mitral commissurotomy is:
- A. Young patient
- B. No history of embolization
- C. Little or no valve calcification
- D. Only moderately severe isolated disease
- E. All of the above

Ref. 4 - p. 2055

B

62. Acute renal failure due to papillary necrosis may be seen most
commonly in patients with:
A. Hyperthyroidism
B. Diabetes mellitus
C. Diabetes insipidus
D. Cushing's syndrome
E. The syndrome of inappro-
priate ADH secretion
Ref. 2 - p. 1147

B

63. The most common factor precipitating convulsions in terminal
renal failure is:
A. Hypokalemia
B. Hypercalcemia
C. Water intoxication
D. Hypophosphatemia
E. Hypermagnesemia
Ref. 2 - p. 1106

E

64. Late effects of head trauma may include:
A. Chronic subdural hematoma
B. Diabetes insipidus
C. Personality changes
D. Seizures
E. All of the above
Ref. 2 - pp. 752, 754-756

A

65. The first symptom of morphine withdrawal generally is:
A. Restlessness
B. Yawning
C. Sweating
D. Muscle cramps and chills
E. Pyrexia
Ref. 2 - p. 588

66. Balance of amniotic fluid is attained mainly by:
A. Control of its production
B. Absorption from fetal membranes
C. Fetal gastrointestinal absorption
D. All of the above
E. None of the above
Ref. 7 - pp. 226-228

67. Hemodialysis may be indicated in the treatment of overdoses of:
A. Bromides
B. Short-acting hypnotics
C. Secobarbital
D. None of the above
E. All of the above
Ref. 2 - p. 605

68. Sulfamylon cream applied to burns may cause:
A. Metabolic acidosis
B. Metabolic alkalosis
C. Respiratory acidosis
D. Respiratory alkalosis
E. None of the above
Ref. 4 - p. 286

C

69. The toxicity of petroleum distillates is related primarily to:
A. Fatty degeneration of the liver
B. Myocardial infarction
C. Aspiration into the respiratory tract
D. Gastric erosion and hemorrhage
E. Pulmonary embolism
Ref. 10 - p. 538

C

70. The most common type of female pelvis is:
A. Anthropoid
B. Android
C. Gynecoid
D. Platypelloid
E. Mixed
Ref. 9 - p. 423

B 71. Which condition is said to improve with pregnancy?
    A. Renal tuberculosis   D. Hepatitis
    B. Sarcoidosis   E. Carcinoma of thyroid
    C. Bronchiectasis   Ref. 7 - p. 788

B 72. Soon after birth, the ductus arteriosus closes because of:
    A. Venturi effect in the aorta
    B. Decreased pulmonary resistance
    C. Increased intraatrial pressure
    D. Spontaneous thrombosis
    E. Rotation of the heart and torsion of the ductus
                              Ref. 6 - p. 716

C 73. Gonadotropins are produced by the _____ of the anterior pituitary:
    A. Basophils   D. Hauptzellen cells
    B. Acidophils   E. None of the above
    C. Chromophobes   Ref. 8 - p. 43

74. In the female embryo, the Wolffian ducts regress after the _____ week.
    A. 7 th   D. 10 th
    B. 8 th   E. 11 th
    C. 9 th   Ref. 8 - p. 132

75. A teenager is on "blue-velvets", that is to say:
    A. Sniffing glue
    B. Injecting a mixture of paregoric and antihistamines
    C. Smoking pot
    D. Injecting heroin
    E. Taking LSD   Ref. 10 - p. 571

76. Sarcoidosis may be associated with cutaneous anergy to:
    A. Tuberculin   D. Mumps virus
    B. Candida albicans   E. All of the above
    C. Trichophyton   Ref. 1 - p. 1061

B 77. High-voltage electrical injuries resemble:
    A. High temperature burns   D. Snakebites
    B. Crush injuries   E. None of the above
    C. Frostbite   Ref. 4 - p. 297

D 78. An oocyte:
    A. Has undergone one meiotic division
    B. Occurs in maximal numbers at 5 months of gestation
    C. Rests in the prophase
    D. All
    E. None   Ref. 8 - p. 130

79. Increased susceptibility to bacterial infections is characteristic of uremia. The factors usually responsible for this may include:
    A. Impaired leukocyte phagocytosis
    B. Delayed appearance of antibodies in response to new antigens
    C. Reduced circulating lymphocytes
    D. All of the above
    E. None of the above   Ref. 2 - p. 1104

80. Chronic ischemia of the foot is recognized early by:
    A. Loss of hair from the toes   D. Skin rubor
    B. Brittle opaque nails   E. All of the above
    C. Skin atrophy   Ref. 6 - p. 840

81. Needle biopsy of the thyroid is contraindicated in:
    A. Hashimoto's thyroiditis   D. Ligneous thyroiditis
    B. Nodular goiter   E. Graves' disease
    C. Carcinoma of the thyroid   Ref. 4 - p. 642

82. Which one of the following is(not)true of Paget's disease of bone?
    A. The disorder is more common in men than women
    B. The disorder commonly involves the weight-bearing bones
    C. There is rapid bone formation and resorption in the involved regions
    D. The serum alkaline phosphatase is always low in this disorder
    E. This disorder frequently predisposes to osteogenic sarcoma
       this is True   Ref. 2 - p. 1842

83. Pulsion diverticulum of the esophagus:
    A. Usually occurs in mid-esophagus
    B. Is caused by pull of extrinsic inflammatory lesion
    C. Is usually small and not clinically significant
    D. Has the neck of sac usually in mid-line
    E. Is a true diverticulum with all esophageal layers present
       Ref. 6 - p. 1018

84. Which one of the following statements regarding carbon monoxide poisoning is not true?
    A. The skin of the victim may be pink
    B. The blood may be cherry red
    C. Vomiting and headaches are common
    D. Patients usually have underlying heart disease
    E. Recovery without sequelae is usual in nonfatal cases
       Ref. 2 - p. 63

85. Which one of the following diseases is most commonly associated with extreme enlargement of the left atrium?
    A. Pulmonary valvular stenosis   D. Ebstein's anomaly
    B. Mitral regurgitation   E. Coarctation of the aorta
    C. Aortic valvular stenosis   Ref. 1 - p. 1190

A 86. ___ % of the population has four parathyroid glands.
    A. 99%   D. 60%
    B. 90%   E. 40%
    C. 80%   Ref. 4 - p. 656

87. A hemorrhage tendency is common in late renal failure. Which one of the following test results is most commonly found in these cases?
    A. Prolonged prothrombin time
    B. Prolonged clotting time
    C. Decreased plasma fibrinogen level
    D. Impaired platelet aggregation with ADP
    E. Shortened euglobulin lysis time   Ref. 2 - p. 1104

88. The primary aim of local burn wound management is to:
    A. Control wound infection
    B. Remove eschar early
    C. Get wound closure and coverage early
    D. Minimize scarring
    E. All of the above   Ref. 4 - p. 282

89. The antibiotic of choice for most infections due to gram-positive bacilli and Neisseria:
    A. Penicillin   D. Chloramphenicol
    B. Erythromycin   E. Polymyxin B
    C. Sulfonamides   Ref. 10 - p. 584

90. Characteristic cerebrospinal fluid findings in viral meningitis:
    A. Cell count may be low
    B. Cell type may be an early polymorphonuclear reaction
    C. Normal sugar content
    D. 1 to 3+ protein
    E. All of the above   Ref. 10 - p. 600

91. The area most likely involved by metastatic spread of an infection from the respiratory tract, caused by H. influenzae:
    A. Pericardial cavity   D. Periorbital region
    B. Anterior cervical lymph nodes E. GI tract
    C. Meninges   Ref. 10 - p. 619

92. Human bites of the face may be sutured primarily, if debrided, within ___ hours of injury, if antibiotics are given.
    A. 2 hours   D. 8 hours
    B. 4 hours   E. Never
    C. 6 hours   Ref. 4 - p. 347

93. Duodenal diverticulum:
    A. Is a rare X-ray finding
    B. Appears on the lateral aspect
    C. May obstruct the common bile duct
    D. Commonly causes duodenal obstruction
    E. Often ulcerates and bleeds   Ref. 6 - p. 1100

C 94. The usual mechanism of ureteral injury is accidental:
A. Instrumental crushing   D. Excision
B. Ligation   E. Puncture
C. Transection   Ref. 4 - p. 1532

E (95.) The maternal mortality rate is defined as:
A. # of maternal deaths/1,000 live births
B. # of maternal deaths/10,000 live births
C. # of maternal deaths/100,000 live births
D. # of maternal deaths/100,000 pregnancies
E. # of maternal deaths/1,000 pregnancies
Ref. 7 - p. 3

C 96. The drug of choice in the treatment of gonorrhea in women is:
A. Oxytetracycline   D. Chloramphenicol
B. Sulfonamides   E. Erythromycin
C. Penicillin   Ref. 9 - p. 498

C 97. All of the following are characteristic of whooping cough, except:
A. Most communicable during catarrhal period
B. Paroxysms of cough may occur after period of contagion
C. Individual susceptibility is great
D. Immunity from mother during first 6 months of life
E. One attack usually confers lasting immunity
Ref. 10 - p. 628

C 98. Streptococcal pharyngitis can be diagnosed with some assurance when:
A. A scarlatiniform rash is present
B. Child exhibits hoarseness, cough and coryza
C. The tonsils are beefy red
D. Fever is high and child vomits
E. Petechiae are found on the soft palate
Ref. 10 - p. 648

A 99. Dimercaprol (BAL) is not useful in the treatment of poisoning due to:
A. Mercury   D. Opium
B. Arsenic   E. Thallium
C. Antimony   Ref. 2 - p. 603

D 100. An erythroderma syndrome may be noted with:
A. Drug reactions   D. All of the above
B. Lymphomas   E. None of the above
C. Psoriasis   Ref. 1 - p. 264

D 101. Post partum inversion of the uterus is seen:
A. With no precipitating causes
B. After Credé removal of the placenta
C. After manual removal of the placenta
D. All of the above
E. None of the above   Ref. 9 - p. 385

A 102. Endometritis post partum is usually produced by:
   A. Streptococcus   D. Pseudomonas
   B. E. coli   E. Proteus
   C. Gonorrhea   Ref. 8 - p. 398

C 103. Hypotension following saddle block anesthesia is due to:
   A. High levels of anesthesia
   B. Obstruction of inferior vena cava
   C. Pooling of blood in the viscera
   D. All of the above
   E. None of the above   Ref. 7 - p. 451

C 104. Morphea refers to:
   A. A localized form of scleroderma
   B. The state of opium addiction
   C. A viral exanthem
   D. Pretibial myxedema
   E. None of the above   Ref. 1 - p. 268

D 105. The nerve so easily injured at repair of patent ductus arteriosus is:
   A. Phrenic   D. Recurrent laryngeal
   B. Vagus trunk   E. Sympathetic trunk
   C. Pulmonary plexus   Ref. 6 - p. 720

E 106. A patient is amenorrheic with well developed breasts, an absent uterus, good estrogen effect on vaginal smear and an absent chromatic body. The most likely diagnosis is:
   A. Turner's syndrome   D. Del-Castilo syndrome
   B. Hypothyroidism   E. Testicular feminization
   C. Chiari-Frommel syndrome   Ref. 8 - pp. 149-150,
                                           173-177

107. Precipitate labor occurs under:
   A. 30 minutes   D. Four hours
   B. One hour   E. Six hours
   C. Two hours   Ref. 9 - p. 362

D 108. All of the following are noted in erythema multiforme except:
   A. Symmetrical distribution   D. Severe toxemia
   B. Crusting of the lips   E. Target lesions
   C. Uniform absence of fever   Ref. 1 - pp. 269, 270

109. True hermaphrodites:
   A. Never menstruate
   B. Are always chromatin positive
   C. Are always XY
   D. Have both testicular and ovarian tissue
   E. None of the above   Ref. 8 - p. 164

β 110. Cystometric studies are of greatest value in identifying:
A. Urge incontinence
B. Neurogenic bladder
C. Fistula
D. Stress incontinence
E. Bladder calculi
Ref. 8 - p. 298

111. "Posterior" chest tubes must not be inserted posterior to:
A. Mid-clavicular line
B. Anterior axillary line
C. Mid-axillary line
D. Posterior axillary line
E. None of the above
Ref. 4 - p. 370

β 112. Bullous lesions of the palms and soles in a two day old child should suggest:
A. Allergy to soap
B. Early congenital syphilis
C. Chickenpox
D. Septicemia with E. coli
E. Milk allergy
Ref. 10 - p. 654

β E 113. Plain X-rays of the skull may show evidence of brain tumor by:
A. Overlying hyperostosis
B. Shift in position of a calcified pineal gland
C. Tumor calcification
D. Erosions such as of sella turcica
E. Any of the above
Ref. 6 - p. 1648

114. A subcapsular hematoma of the spleen secondary to blunt trauma should be treated by:
A. Splenectomy
B. Careful observation for 48 hours
C. Observation for 7 days
D. Observation for 10-14 days
E. Observation for a minimum of 3 weeks
Ref. 4 - p. 381

115. In first degree hypospadias, the most frequent complication is:
A. Penile-scrotal angle fistula
B. Chordee
C. Dorsal curvature
D. Bifid scrotum
E. Short urethra
Ref. 6 - p. 1963

116. Pruritus may be associated with:
A. Hyperthyroidism
B. Pregnancy
C. Polycythemia vera
D. All of the above
E. None of the above
Ref. 1 - p. 272

117. The most common syndrome associated with benign adrenal cortical adenoma is:
A. Adrenal virilism
B. Primary aldosteronism
C. Cushing's syndrome
D. All of the above
E. None of the above
Ref. 6 - p. 1395

118. Plain X-ray films of the skull after head injury may be helpful in showing:
   A. Displaced calcified pineal gland
   B. Depressed fracture
   C. Fracture line crossing arterial groove
   D. Air in the cranial cavity
   E. Any of the above   Ref. 6 - p. 1636

119. Withdrawal bleeding due to progesterone administration means:
   A. Estrogen is present in sufficient quantity
   B. There is no ovarian failure
   C. An intact endometrium
   D. All of the above
   E. None of the above   Ref. 8 - p. 700

120. Melatonin is a hormone secreted by the:
   A. Anterior pituitary gland   D. Sympathetic ganglia in the
   B. Pineal gland   thoracic region
   C. Hypothalamus   E. Posterior pituitary gland
                                        Ref. 1 - p. 587

121. Gynecomastia may be seen in patients with:
   A. Klinefelter's syndrome   D. Cirrhosis of the liver
   B. Digitalis therapy   E. All of the above
   C. Aldactone therapy   Ref. 1 - p. 583

122. The greatest increase of the SGOT occurs in:
   A. Myocardial infarction   D. Angina pectoris
   B. Idiopathic pericarditis   E. All of the above
   C. Rheumatic carditis   Ref. 1 - p. 1518

123. Ureteral injuries most often are a result of:
   A. Blunt abdominal trauma   D. Gunshot wounds of the ab-
   B. Stab wounds of the abdomen   domen
   C. Stab wounds of the flank   E. Surgical trauma
                                        Ref. 4 - p. 1523

124. Approximately ____ % of the gas that distends the small intestine is the result of swallowed air.
   A. 90%   D. 25%
   B. 70%   E. Less than 10%
   C. 50%   Ref. 4 - p. 409

125. A pellagra-like skin rash may be observed as a complication of therapy with:
   A. INH   D. Streptomycin
   B. PAS   E. None of the above
   C. Cycloserine   Ref. 1 - p. 429

126. With regard to precocious puberty:
   A. It includes both menstruation and secondary sexual develop-
      ment before age 12
   B. May be caused by thalamic tumors
   C. Never is idiopathic
   D. All of the above
   E. None of the above   Ref. 8 - pp. 703-706

127. If several ribs are fractured both anteriorly and posteriorly,
    early death most often is due to:
   A. Pneumonia   D. Lung collapse
   B. Flail chest   E. Emphysema
   C. Hemothorax   Ref. 4 - p. 371

128. The segment of bowel most susceptible to tension gangrene has:
   A. Thin wall, large diameter   D. Thick wall, small diameter
   B. Thin wall, small diameter   E. These are not relevant fac-
   C. Thick wall, large diameter   tors
                              Ref. 6 - p. 983

129. A strong relationship has been demonstrated between ultra-
    violet radiation and:
   A. Basal-cell carcinoma   D. Multiple myeloma
   B. Sarcoidosis   E. Multiple sclerosis
   C. Lupus erythematosus   Ref. 1 - p. 283

130. Manifestations of anemia frequently include all of the following
    except:
   A. Tinnitus   D. Headache
   B. Restlessness   E. Vertigo
   C. Delirium   Ref. 1 - p. 295

131. The principal component of the system which protects the
    red blood cell and its contents from oxidation is:
   A. Glutathione
   B. Reduced triphosphopyridine nucleotide (TPNH, NADPH)
   C. The enzyme glucose 6-phosphate dehydrogenase
   D. The enzymes glutathione reductase and glutathione peroxi-
      dase
   E. All of the above   Ref. 1 - pp. 1602-1607

132. In renal transplants, "warm ischemia time" in excess of
    _____ minutes is undesirable, but still acceptable.
   A. 5 minutes   D. 30 minutes
   B. 10 minutes   E. 60 minutes
   C. 15 minutes   Ref. 4 - p. 453

133. In iron deficiency anemia:
   A. The serum iron-binding capacity is decreased
   B. The marrow iron stores are normal
   C. The sideroblasts in the marrow are increased
   D. The serum iron concentration is decreased
   E. All of the above   Ref. 1 - p. 1583

134. Inguinal lymphadenitis rarely occurs with:
     A. Lymphopathia venereum
     B. Granuloma inguinale
     C. Chancroid
     D. Syphilitic chancre
     E. None of the above
        Ref. 8 - p. 188

135. The fetal origin of the placenta begins with the:
     A. Decidua basalis
     B. Decidua spongiosa
     C. Decidua vera
     D. Chorion frondosum
     E. Chorion laeve
        Ref. 7 - pp. 143-149

136. Chorionic Somatomammotropin:
     A. Cross reacts with LH
     B. Depresses the level of circulating free fatty levels
     C. Depresses maternal insulin levels
     D. Inhibits gluconeogenesis
     E. None
        Ref. 7 - p. 176

137. If an Rh negative multigravida with a Rh positive husband develops hydramnios at 36 weeks gestation, one should:
     A. Treat the patient expectantly
     B. Do an Rh antibody titre on the mother
     C. Perform an amniocentesis to get fluid for spectrophotometric examination
     D. Induce labor
     E. None of the above
        Ref. 9 - p. 390

138. The majority of hemoglobin in erythrocytes from normal adults is termed:
     A. Hemoglobin F
     B. Hemoglobin A_2
     C. Hemoglobin Bart's
     D. Hemoglobin A
     E. Hemoblogin C
        Ref. 1 - p. 1614

139. The major cause of maternal mortality from obstetrical anesthesia is:
     A. Respiratory failure
     B. Cardiac standstill
     C. Aspiration of vomitus
     D. Fatal reaction to local anesthetic
     E. Hemorrhage and shock
        Ref. 7 - p. 786

140. Laboratory data in sideroblastic anemia include:
     A. Increased serum iron
     B. Decreased serum iron-binding capacity
     C. Increased iron stores in the marrow
     D. Increased marrow sideroblasts
     E. All of the above
        Ref. 1 - p. 297

141. The physiological retraction ring is identical with:
     A. The anatomic internal cervical os
     B. The histological internal cervical os
     C. Bandl's ring
     D. The uterine isthmus
     E. All of the above
        Ref. 7 - p. 850

142. The myeloid/erythroid ratio is decreased in all of the following except:
   A. Iron-deficiency anemia
   B. Sideroblastic anemia
   C. The majority of infections
   D. Thalassemia
   E. Cirrhosis of the liver
   Ref. 1 - p. 298

143. A breech hydrocephalus may be managed by:
   A. Cesarean section
   B. Destructive procedure
   C. Decompression of the head transvaginally
   D. Decompression of the head transabdominally
   E. All of the above
   Ref. 7 - pp. 885-888

144. Which of the following is not true of treatment of duodenal fistula?
   A. Naso-duodenal suction is important
   B. Tract should be kept empty and dry by sump drainage
   C. Skin should be protected from chemical erosion
   D. Immediate operative closure is advised
   E. Jejunostomy tube for feeding may be needed
   Ref. 6 - p. 485

145. A malignant melanoma should be excised with a margin of at least _____ cm in each direction.
   A. 1 cm
   B. 2 cm
   C. 5 cm
   D. 7 cm
   E. 9 cm
   Ref. 4 - p. 566

146. Adequate fern pattern from drying cervical mucus suggests adequate output of:
   A. Progesterone
   B. 17-ketosteroids
   C. Cholesterol
   D. Estrogen
   E. 17-hydroxycorticosteroids
   Ref. 6 - p. 1595

147. The chemotherapeutic agent used in Wilms' tumor is:
   A. Fluorouracil
   B. Actinomycin D
   C. Chlorambucil
   D. Busulfan
   E. Cytoxan
   Ref. 4 - p. 1196

148. A bloody nipple discharge is usually associated with:
   A. Lactation
   B. Early pregnancy
   C. Galactocele
   D. Intraductal papilloma
   E. Fibroadenoma
   Ref. 4 - p. 574

149. The most common form of cancer in women in the U.S. is:
   A. Breast
   B. Lung
   C. Cervix
   D. Ovary
   E. Colon
   Ref. 4 - p. 580

150. Pes cavus most frequently is a result of:
    A. Myelodysplasia
    B. Spina bifida
    C. Muscular dystrophy
    D. Poliomyelitis
    E. Idiopathic causes
       Ref. 6 - p. 1699

151. Features of a case of drug poisoning with LSD might include all of the following except:
    A. Confusion
    B. Panic
    C. Dilated pupils
    D. Phenothiazine treatment as drug treatment of choice
    E. Hyperreflexia
       Ref. 2 - p. 603

152. The mortality in patients with ruptured uterus is:
    A. Higher in the mother
    B. Higher in the fetus
    C. Same in the mother and fetus
    D. Lower in the fetus
    E. None of the above
       Ref. 7 - pp. 936-956

153. Regarding scalene fat pad biopsy:
    A. Damage to phrenic nerve is a real danger
    B. 25% positive in cases of lung cancer
    C. Damage to the thoracic duct is a distinct possibility
    D. 80% positive in cases of Boeck's sarcoid
    E. All of the above are true
       Ref. 6 - p. 649

154. Which one of the following statements regarding psittacosis is true?
    A. It is almost always transmitted to man by the respiratory route
    B. Cold agglutinins are commonly present in high titres
    C. Piperazine citrate is effective in severe cases
    D. Headache is almost never a complaint
    E. Tetracycline is generally ineffective in treatment
       Ref. 1 - p. 941

155. In the United States, carcinoma of the _____ is undergoing the greatest decline in incidence:
    A. Esophagus
    B. Stomach
    C. Pancreas
    D. Liver
    E. Colon
       Ref. 2 - p. 1294

156. Which one of the following lesions is commonly found in the posterior mediastinum?
    A. Substernal thyroid adenoma
    B. Dermoid cyst
    C. Neurofibroma
    D. Teratoma
    E. Thymoma
       Ref. 1 - p. 1330

157. Concerning the tuberculin reaction:
    A. A positive reaction to tuberculin indicates the presence of allergy to tuberculin and the presence of tuberculous infection
    B. A positive tuberculin test is expected among BCG-vaccinated individuals

C. A negative test may occur in a person in the incubation
   period
D. All of the above
E. None of the above   Ref. 10 - p. 682

158. A child with proven cat scratch disease should:
    A. Receive a therapeutic trial of penicillin
    B. Be desensitized with allergen
    C. Have surgical removal of enlarged nodes
    D. All of the above
    E. None of the above   Ref. 10 - p. 699

159. All of the following are characteristic of rabies, except:
    A. Usually transmitted by bites of dogs, cats, bats and wild
       animals
    B. Rabies virus is resistant to commonly used skin antiseptics
    C. Virus usually cannot be introduced through intact skin
    D. Incubation period is short: 2 to 5 days
    E. Negri bodies are pathognomonic features of rabies infection
                                       Ref. 10 - pp. 755-756

160. The average incubation period for Rocky Mountain spotted fever
    is:
    A. 2 days   D. 21 days
    B. 7 days   E. 3 months
    C. 14 days   Ref. 10 - p. 781

161. The drug of choice in the treatment of trigeminal neuralgia is:
    A. Chlorpromazine   D. Morphine
    B. Phenobarbital   E. Aspirin
    C. Carbamazepine   Ref. 2 - p. 612

162. Regarding adrenal cortical carcinomas, which statement is
    false:
    A. 17 ketosteroids are elevated
    B. Most are functional
    C. Patients may present with Cushing's syndrome
    D. Posterior surgical approach is preferred
    E. Blood pressure may be elevated   Ref. 4 - p. 696

163. Each of the following is characteristic of cystic fibrosis of the
    pancreas, except:
    A. Meconium ileus   D. Common in Negroes
    B. Chronic pulmonary infection E. Malnutrition and shortened
    C. Pancreatic insufficiency   stature
                                   Ref. 2 - p. 1252

164. Trigeminal neuralgia is sometimes associated with:
    A. Syringomyelia
    B. Amyotrophic lateral sclerosis
    C. Subacute combined degeneration of the cord
    D. Reye's syndrome
    E. Multiple sclerosis   Ref. 2 - p. 612

165. Each of the following findings may be commonly observed in aplastic anemia, except:
    A. Indolent ulcers in the mouth
    B. Usually normal blood coagulation
    C. Marked splenomegaly
    D. Usually elevated serum iron
    E. Very low reticulocyte count   Ref. 2 - p. 1417

166. The following statements about hidradenitis suppurativa are true, except:
    A. In early cases, improved hygiene, incision and drainage, are adequate
    B. Local antibiotic creams will control the infection at any stage
    C. X-ray therapy is effective in early cases
    D. In chronic cases, total skin excision and grafting is required
    E. Mixed saprophytes, streptococci and staphylococci are the cause   Ref. 6 - p. 516

167. The symptoms of vitamin A excess include all of the following, except:
    A. Anorexia   D. Congestive heart failure
    B. Hair loss   E. Bone demineralization
    C. Headache   Ref. 1 - p. 439

168. Regarding left to right shunts, all are true, except:
    A. Left heart pressures normally exceed those on the right
    B. Cyanosis is a prominent feature
    C. Oxygenated blood is shunted from left to right
    D. Pulmonary congestion is a prominent feature
    E. Systemic flow is decreased   Ref. 6 - p. 679

169. All are causes of post spinal headache, except:
    A. Dehydration
    B. Altered cerebrospinal fluid pressure
    C. Rapid change in blood volume post delivery
    D. Early ambulation   Ref. 9 - p. 373

170. One of the principal intracranial pain-sensitive structures is:
    A. The cranium
    B. The brain parenchyma
    C. The ependymal lining of the ventricles
    D. Most of the dura
    E. None of the above   Ref. 2 - p. 614

171. During rigid esophagoscopy, the area of the esophagus most often perforated is:
    A. At the cricopharyngeus muscle
    B. At the aortic arch
    C. At the mid-esophagus
    D. At the esophago-gastric junction
    E. None of the above   Ref. 4 - p. 742

172. Electrical cardioversion is a useful mode of therapy in each of the following, except:
    A. Ventricular tachycardia
    B. Atrial fibrillation
    C. Ventricular fibrillation
    D. Atrial flutter
    E. Bradycardia due to hypo-thyroidism
    Ref. 1 - p. 1152

173. The following statements about testicular tumor are true, except:
    A. Chorioepithelioma metastasizes by the blood stream
    B. Seminoma is highly radio-sensitive
    C. Retroperitoneal node involvement is limited by the diaphragm
    D. Tumors are hard, irregular, painless and heavy
    E. Lymphography shows adequacy of node dissection
    Ref. 4 - p. 1567

174. Disorders of coagulation are characterized by all of the following except:
    A. Hemarthrosis
    B. Delayed bleeding
    C. Superficial ecchymoses
    D. 80% occurrence of heredi-tary disorders in females
    E. Absence of petechiae
    Ref. 1 - p. 305

175. _____ % of duodenal ulcers occur in the duodenal bulb.
    A. 95%
    B. 75%
    C. 50%
    D. 25%
    E. 10%
    Ref. 4 - p. 830

176. Each of the following statements about carcinoma of the colon in patients with ulcerative colitis is true, except:
    A. Carcinoma of the colon tends to be increased in incidence
    B. The carcinoma is often multicentric in origin
    C. Risk of carcinoma is greatest in those patients with late on-set of disease
    D. Risk of carcinoma is high in patients with widespread di-sease
    E. Carcinoma is most common in the rectosigmoid area
    Ref. 2 - p. 1270

177. All are associated with CNS injury to newborn, except:
    A. Narcosis
    B. Hypoxia
    C. Brain damage
    D. Acidosis
    E. Alkalosis
    Ref. 7 - pp. 1009-1020

178. All of the following are causes of mechanical intestinal ob-struction, except:
    A. Inflammatory adhesions
    B. Adynamic ileus of peritonitis
    C. Gallstone obturation
    D. Intussusception
    E. Extrinsic tumor pressure
    Ref. 6 - p. 980

179. Slowly developing ataxia is associated with all of the following, except:
   A. Cerebellar tumors
   B. Heredodegenerative disorders
   C. Varicella
   D. Hartnup disease
   E. Brainstem tumors   Ref. 10 - p. 851

180. The features of long-standing sickle cell anemia in an adult may include each of the following, except:
   A. Hematuria
   B. Aseptic necrosis of bones
   C. Impaired ability to concentrate urine
   D. Chronic leg ulcers
   E. Massive splenomegaly   Ref. 1 - p. 1620

181. In Cushing's adrenocortical syndrome, positive laboratory findings include all, except:
   A. Hypoglycemia   D. Leukocytosis
   B. Decreased glucose tolerance   E. Increased urinary excre-
   C. Eosinopenia   tion of corticosteroids
                                     Ref. 6 - p. 1383

182. The treatment of digitalis-induced arrhythmias may include each of the following, except:
   A. Potassium supplements
   B. Withdrawal of digitalis
   C. Lidocaine administration
   D. Calcium gluconate administration
   E. Diphenylhydantoin administration
                                     Ref. 1 - p. 1146

183. In bleeding caused by thrombocytopenia:
   A. Petechiae are frequently noted
   B. Deep dissecting hematomas are common
   C. Hemarthroses are common
   D. Delayed bleeding is noted frequently
   E. None of the above   Ref. 1 - p. 305

184. All of the following statements regarding Wilms' tumor are correct, except:
   A. Proper therapy before age 2 gives a 73% survival rate
   B. Osseous and pulmonary metastases decrease effectiveness of chemotherapy
   C. Proper therapy after age 2 gives 18% survival rate
   D. About 5% of Wilms' tumors are bilateral
   E. Proper therapy is chemotherapy and irradiation followed by nephrectomy   Ref. 6 - p. 1567

185. Each of the following is suggestive of regional enteritis, except:
    A. Lower right abdominal pain
    B. Perirectal fistulas
    C. Abdominal pain
    D. Increased incidence of gastric cancer
    E. Diarrhea
    Ref. 2 - p. 1258

186. Each of the following statements regarding the acute radiation syndrome is usually true, except:
    A. Nausea and vomiting are common
    B. Patients often enter a phase of relative well being after the initial symptoms
    C. Marked lymphocytosis characteristically occurs early in illness
    D. Loss of the scalp hair may occur
    E. Bone marrow suppression may occur
    Ref. 2 - p. 68

187. All of the following are true of face presentations, except:
    A. X-ray pelvimetry is essential to rule out pelvic contraction
    B. If pelvis is normal the chin anterior vaginal delivery should be anticipated
    C. If pelvis is normal the chin posterior spontaneous rotation should occur in about 2/3 of cases
    D. Manual conversion to a vertex should always be attempted
    E. Version and extraction should be attempted in women with normal pelvis
    Ref. 7 - pp. 863-870

188. As many as ____ % of gastric carcinomas may pass a 12 week trial of healing.
    A. 75%
    B. 50%
    C. 33%
    D. 16%
    E. 8%
    Ref. 4 - p. 840

Each group of questions below consists of lettered headings followed by a list of numbered words or phrases. For each numbered word or phrase select the one heading which is most closely related to it:

Match item with type of rib tumor:

    A. Fibrous dysplasia
    B. Eosinophilic granuloma
    C. Ewing's sarcoma
    D. Myeloma
    E. Hyperparathyroidism

189. ____ Multiple osteolytic areas without osteogenesis
190. ____ Onion-skin calcification
191. ____ Demineralization and cystic lesions
192. ____ Excise to distinguish from malignancy
193. ____ Swelling over punched-out osteolytic lesion
    Ref. 6 - p. 606

Match the following:

A. Familial polyposis
B. Juvenile polyposis
C. Gardner's syndrome
D. Peutz-Jeghers syndrome

194. ___ Associated with melanin spots on buccal mucosa
195. ___ Occurs at very early age and is not premalignant
196. ___ Premalignant polyps, osteomas, soft tissue tumors
197. ___ Premalignant and rarely seen before puberty
198. ___ Polyps are considered hamartomas
                                        Ref. 4 - pp. 984-987

A. Increased incidence in hemochromatosis
B. Possible association with Plummer-Vinson syndrome
C. Increased frequency in ulcerative colitis
D. Migratory thrombophlebitis
E. Decreasing in frequency

199. ___ Carcinoma of the colon
200. ___ Carcinoma of the stomach
201. ___ Carcinoma of the pancreas
202. ___ Carcinoma of the esophagus
203. ___ Carcinoma of the liver   Ref. 2 - pp. 1270, 1294,
                                                1254, 1291,
                                                1352

A. Treacher-Collins syndrome
B. Pierre Robin syndrome
C. Silver syndrome
D. Cornelia de Lange syndrome
E. Hallerman-Streiff syndrome

204. ___ Micrognathia, glossoptosis, cleft palate
205. ___ Continuous eyebrows, hirsutism, short stature, mental deficiency, small or malformed hands and feet
206. ___ Triangular hypoplastic facies, skeletal asymmetry, clinodactyly of fifth finger, short stature
207. ___ Malar and mandibular hypoplasia, defect of lower eyelid, malformation of external ear
208. ___ Hypotrichosis, short stature, microphthalmia and cataracts, micrognathia   Ref. 11 - pp. 1701-1702

Match location of radial shaft fracture with fragment displacement:

A. Pronation
B. Supination
C. Mid-position
D. Ulnar deviation

209. ___ Above pronator, proximal fragment
210. ___ Above pronator, distal fragment
211. ___ Below pronator, proximal fragment
212. ___ Below pronator, distal fragment
213. ___ Lower shaft   Ref. 4 - p. 1339

A. Clindamycin
B. Tetracycline
C. Gentamycin
D. Sulfisoxazole
E. Chloramphenicol

214. ___ Drug of choice for typhoid fever
215. ___ Excellent drug for Mycoplasma
216. ___ One of the best drugs for Bacteroides fragilis
217. ___ Severe renal and vestibular damage
218. ___ May cause erythema multiforme and hemolytic anemia
                                    Ref. 1 - pp. 746-748

A. Poisoning with carbon monoxide
B. Poisoning with cleaning solutions
C. Poisoning with chlorinated insecticides
D. Poisoning with digitalis
E. Poisoning with cyanide

219. ___ Hyperexcitability, tremors, ataxia, convulsions, followed by CNS depression, epinephrine is contraindicated
220. ___ Severe headache, weakness, dizziness, nausea, vomiting, collapse, coma, failing respirations, cherry red color of lips and fingernails
221. ___ Detergents, halogenated hydrocarbons, sodium sulfate
222. ___ Giddiness, hyperpnea, headache, palpitation, cyanosis, unconsciousness, asphyxial convulsions, death in a few seconds to minutes
223. ___ Arrhythmias, bradycardia, drowsiness, coma, death from ventricular fibrillation   Ref. 11 - pp. 1668-1670

A. Subhyaloid hemorrhage
B. Thalamic hemorrhage
C. Brainstem hemorrhage
D. Cerebellar hemorrhage
E. Capsular hemorrhage

224. ___ Paralysis of upward gaze frequently noted
225. ___ Seen commonly in subarachnoid hemorrhages
226. ___ Occipital headache, nystagmus and ataxia
227. ___ Loss of consciousness, irregular breathing and pinpoint pupils
228. ___ Homonymous hemianopsia, flaccid paralysis and sensory perception loss which develop rapidly
                                    Ref. 2 - pp. 665, 666

Match the following:

A. Indirect inguinal hernia
B. Direct inguinal hernia
C. Umbilical hernia
D. Femoral hernia
E. Spigelian hernia

229. ___ Occurs at lateral edge of rectus muscle
230. ___ Often closes by age 2
231. ___ More common in blacks than in whites
232. ___ Lateral to inferior epigastric vessels
233. ___ Medial to inferior epigastric vessels

Ref. 4 - pp. 1153-1163

Match the following:

A. Fetal death
B. Isthmic softening of cervix
C. Venous engorgement of vagina
D. Discoloration of periumbilical skin
E. Calf tenderness

234. ___ Chadwick's sign
235. ___ Hegar's sign
236. ___ Spalding's sign
237. ___ Homans' sign
238. ___ Cullen's sign

Ref. 7 - pp. 245, 281, 289,
547, 1002

A. Waardenburg's syndrome
B. 18-trisomy syndrome
C. Familial dysautonomia
D. Marfan's syndrome
E. Down syndrome (21-trisomy)

239. ___ Blepharophimosis, congenital deafness, white forelock
240. ___ Epicanthus, Brushfield spots, cataracts, simian crease, clindodactyly
241. ___ Ptosis, epicanthal folds, strabismus, fish-like mouth, flexion deformities of fingers, prominent occiput
242. ___ Subluxated lenses, arachnodactyly, kyphoscoliosis, laxity of joints
243. ___ Deficiency of tears, corneal anesthesia, corneal ulcers, pupillary miosis with methacholine 2.5%

Ref. 11 - pp. 1098, 1692,
1699, 1704

A. Actinomycosis
B. Cryptococcosis
C. Aspergillosis
D. Mycoplasma
E. Pneumocystis carinii

244. ___ Pentamidine isethionate
245. ___ Thrombosis of pulmonary vessels by invading mycelia
246. ___ Encapsulated yeast seen well with India ink stain
247. ___ Gram-positive filamentous organism
248. ___ Cold agglutinin-positive pneumonia

Ref. 1 - pp. 1032, 906, 896, 894, 936

Match operation with indication for its use:

A. Sphincterotomy
B. Anastomosis to stomach
C. Whipple pancreaticoduodenal resection
D. Lay open duct and anastomose side-to-side with jejunum
E. Caudal pancreatojejunostomy

249. ___ Pseudocyst
250. ___ Stone-obstructed pancreatic duct
251. ___ Multiple pancreatic duct obstructions
252. ___ Mild disease with obstruction at papilla
253. ___ Chronic pancreatitis of the head with common bile duct
stenosis   Ref. 6 - pp. 1263-1270

For each numbered word or phrase select the correct answer by using the key outlined below:

A. If the item is associated with A only
B. If the item is associated with B only
C. If the item is associated with both A and B
D. If the item is associated with neither A nor B

A. Ampullary pregnancy
B. Interstitial pregnancy
C. Both
D. Neither

254. ___ A mass is palpable
255. ___ May give rise to uterine asymmetry
256. ___ Rupture may result in exsanguination in one hour
257. ___ Rupture may occur during the second trimester
258. ___ May result in tubal abortion

Ref. 7 - pp. 541; 551-552

A. Ollier's disease (chondrodysplasia)
B. Arthrogryposis
C. Both
D. Neither

259. ___ Usually unilateral, facial asymmetry
260. ___ Inherited as an autosomal recessive
261. ___ Gradual onset during first few years of life
262. ___ Elbows and knees usually ankylosed in extension
263. ___ Treatment with corticosteroids is initial program

Ref. 11 - pp. 1486-1489

   A. Duodenal ulcer
   B. Marginal ulcer
   C. Both
   D. Neither

264. ___ Vagotomy is good treatment
265. ___ Anemia more prominent than hematemesis
266. ___ Perforation into colon is not uncommon
267. ___ Greater tendency to complications
268. ___ Due to Zollinger-Ellison tumor in some cases
                                    Ref. 6 - pp. 1055-1069

   A. Choriocarcinoma of testis
   B. Seminoma
   C. Both
   D. Neither

269. ___ Highly radiosensitive
270. ___ Most highly fatal of all testicular tumors
271. ___ Radical retroperitoneal node dissection advised
272. ___ Retroperitoneal irradiation advised
273. ___ Orchiectomy alone is sufficient
                                    Ref. 4 - pp. 1565-1567

   A. Aortic valvular stenosis
   B. Aortic regurgitation
   C. Both
   D. Neither

274. ___ Almost never due to syphilis
275. ___ "Water hammer" pulse may be present
276. ___ Angina may occur
277. ___ When heart failure occurs digitalis is contraindicated
278. ___ Associated with Marfan's syndrome
                                    Ref. 1 - pp. 1178-1179,
                                                1182

In fractures of tibial or femoral condyles:

   A. Tibial condyles
   B. Femoral condyles
   C. Both
   D. Neither

279. ___ Popliteal artery injury
280. ___ Tibial nerve injury
281. ___ Peroneal nerve injury
282. ___ Traumatic arthritis of hip, knee or ankle
283. ___ Collateral and cruciate ligament injury
                                    Ref. 6 - pp. 1825-1829

A. Adrenal cortical carcinoma
B. Adrenal cortical hyperplasia
C. Both
D. Neither

284. ___ May have increased plasma ACTH levels
285. ___ Supression of urine 17-hydroxycorticoid excretion after 8 mgs of dexamethasone daily for 3 days
286. ___ No significant increase in urinary 17-hydroxycorticoid excretion following ACTH stimulation
287. ___ May be associated with carcinoma of the bronchus
288. ___ Hypokalemic alkalosis may occur
Ref. 1 - p. 498

A. Idiopathic thrombocytopenic purpura
B. Wiskott-Aldrich syndrome
C. Both
D. Neither

289. ___ Eczema, thrombocytopenic hemorrhage, increased susceptibility to infections
290. ___ Transmitted as an autosomal recessive
291. ___ Splenectomy when patient does not respond to corticosteroids
292. ___ Bone marrow contains normal number of megakaryocytes or increased number
293. ___ Corticosteroids of great value in therapy
Ref. 11 - pp. 1156-1157

A. Smallpox
B. Chickenpox
C. Both
D. Neither

294. ___ Encephalomyelitis
295. ___ Nodular pulmonary calcification
296. ___ Herpes zoster
297. ___ Highly contagious
298. ___ Vaccination is in widespread use
Ref. 1 - pp. 966,969

A. Open mitral valve operation
B. Closed digital commissurotomy
C. Both
D. Neither

299. ___ Best after cerebral embolization
300. ___ Usually physiologically satisfactory
301. ___ Dangerous with extensive calcification
302. ___ Best in recurrent cases
303. ___ Regurgitation cannot be corrected
Ref. 4 - p. 2054

A. Obstructive pulmonary disease
B. Restrictive pulmonary disease
C. Both
D. Neither

304. ___ Bronchial asthma
305. ___ Hamman-Rich syndrome
306. ___ Bagassosis
307. ___ Hypoxemia
308. ___ Pulmonary sarcoidosis   Ref. 1 - pp. 372, 1336,
                                              1309, 1060

After each of the following case histories there is a series of multiple choice questions based on the history. Select the one most appropriate answer:

CASE (Questions 309-312): A 75-year-old woman has a 2 cm ulcerative lesion near the clitoris. Biopsy shows it to be an invasive carcinoma.

309. The most likely histologic picture is that of:
     A. Adenocarcinoma   D. Bowen's disease
     B. Paget's disease   E. Basal cell carcinoma
     C. Squamous cell carcinoma   Ref. 8 - p. 204

310. The lymphatic drainage of the vulva is such that invasive cancer spreads first to:
     A. External iliac nodes   D. Obturator nodes
     B. Femoral nodes   E. Hypogastric nodes
     C. Superficial inguinal nodes   Ref. 8 - p. 204

311. The lesion which predisposes to vulvar cancer in young patients:
     A. Leukoplakia   D. Hidradenoma
     B. Granuloma inguinale   E. None of the above
     C. Syphilis   Ref. 8 - p. 188

312. Which of the following is not true about vulvar cancer therapy?
     A. Radiation is not the preferred method of treatment
     B. Vulvar cancer is relatively radioresistant
     C. Vulva tolerates radiation very poorly
     D. Superficial node dissection and vulvectomy is the best treatment
     E. None of the above   Ref. 8 - p. 207

CASE (Questions 313-316): A 38-year-old housewife noticed increasing fatigue with severe dyspnea on climbing one flight of stairs. Recently she had a chronic cough and was unable to sleep flat in bed. There had been some transient psychic changes with some muscle weakness in the right arm. There was a diastolic rumble near the cardiac apex.

313. Additionally, one might expect to find:
   A. Collapsed neck veins   D. Calcified pericardium
   B. Apical pulmonary rales   E. None of the above
   C. Small cardiac silhouette

314. X-ray examination in this case of mitral stenosis may show:
   A. Left atrial displacement of the mid-esophagus
   B. Straightening of the left cardiac border
   C. Mitral valve calcification
   D. Engorged pulmonary veins
   E. All of the above

315. The transient psychic changes and muscle weakness in the arm make you suspect:
   A. Repeated small embolization   D. Increasing valve stenosis
   B. Polycythemia   E. Beginning regurgitation
   C. Cerebral arteriosclerosis

316. In this case, at operation it is important to:
   A. Open the valve as widely as possible
   B. Flush all clots out of the atrium before opening the valve
   C. Remove all calcium deposits from the leaflets
   D. Use a valvulotomy rather than finger commissurotomy
   E. Shorten the papillary muscles to prevent regurgitation
   Ref. 6 - pp. 762-766

CASE (Questions 317-320): A 54-year-old male complained of the sudden onset of severe left anterior chest pain radiating to the left arm. The pain was not relieved by nitroglycerine tablets. The patient was markedly short of breath and expectorating blood-tinged frothy sputum. The skin was cold, cyanotic and clammy. BP 80/60 mm Hg; heart rate was 120/min and regular. He was oliguric. Examination of the lungs revealed diffuse wheezing and crepitant rales bilaterally. The heart sounds were soft and no murmurs were heard. A third heart sound was heard at the apex.

317. This patient is most probably suffering from:
   A. Dissecting aneurysm
   B. Acute pulmonary edema secondary to myocardial infarction
   C. Acute viral pneumonia with pleuritic chest pain
   D. Acute bronchial asthma
   E. Acute bronchial asthma with angina pectoris

318. The drug most often useful in the treatment of this condition is:
   A. Epinephrine   D. Aspirin
   B. Insulin   E. Tetracycline
   C. Morphine

319. This patient is most likely to have:
    A. Metabolic alkalosis
    B. Bronchiectasis
    C. Metabolic acidosis
    D. Pheochromocytoma
    E. Alpha cell tumor of the pancreas

320. The mortality rate in patients with cardiogenic shock is approximately:
    A. 10%
    B. 30%
    C. 65%
    D. 85%
    E. 100%
    Ref. 2 - pp. 1008, 890, 1013

CASE (Questions 321-324): A newborn boy had a soft, fluctuant, lobulated mass on the posterior neck, extending into the right axilla. It transilluminated well.

321. The diagnosis in this case is:
    A. Cystic hygroma
    B. Branchial cleft cyst
    C. Spring-water cyst
    D. Esophageal duplication cyst
    E. Myelocele

322. The following statements regarding this lesion are true, except:
    A. It is multilocular, thin walled, endothelial lined and lymph filled
    B. Causes the head to be held to the opposite side
    C. It tends to grow and extend
    D. The child must attain the age of three before operation can be undertaken
    E. Without early treatment, the mediastinum may become involved

323. The reason for early treatment is:
    A. Severe spontaneous infection is common
    B. Hemorrhage into the cyst may be fatal
    C. The lesion is unsightly and deforming
    D. Respiratory obstruction may result
    E. All of the above

324. Preferred treatment is:
    A. Injection of sclerosing solution
    B. Pressure dressings
    C. Radical surgical excision
    D. X-ray therapy
    E. Cortisone administration
    Ref. 6 - p. 1515

CASE (Questions 325-328): A young primigravida develops a persistent transverse position of the vertex.

325. Persistent transverse position has the poorest prognosis in:
    A. Gynecoid pelvis
    B. Android pelvis
    C. Anthropoid pelvis
    D. Platypelloid pelvis
    E. All of the above

326. In this type of pelvis the head descends in which position?
   A. Anterior asynclitism
   B. Posterior asynclitism
   C. Synclitic
   D. All of the above
   E. None of the above

327. Failure of anterior rotation of the vertex occurs if:
   A. There is a decreased posterior diameter of the outlet
   B. There is an enlarged mid-pelvis
   C. The AP diameter of the inlet is smaller than the transverse diameter
   D. All of the above
   E. None of the above

328. Characteristic of this type of pelvis is:
   A. Wedge shaped inlet
   B. Sacrosciatic notch is wide
   C. Wide retropubic angle
   D. Sacrum is curved
   E. Side wall of pelvis are straight
   Ref. 9 - p. 430

CASE (Questions 329-332): A 200 pound 67-year-old woman slipped on the ice and fell heavily on the sidewalk, landing on the lateral aspect of her right hip. She was able to walk with pain. This increased over the next three days. Aside from an extensive ecchymosis over the right hip, pain on motion at the hip and a suggestion that the left leg was about two centimeters longer than its mate, findings were negative.

329. X-ray of the hips showed which on the right?
   A. Impacted femoral neck fracture in good position
   B. Complete displacement of the femoral head fracture
   C. Varus position of the femoral head fragment
   D. Valgus position with femoral head tilted posteriorly
   E. Intertrochanteric fracture

330. Since the head was in valgus position, impacted upon the neck, without anterior or posterior neck-head displacement, treatment could be by:
   A. Primary cast application
   B. Skeletal traction
   C. Non-weight-bearing without immobilization or fixation
   D. Smith-Petersen nail
   E. Choice of any of the above

331. The doctor decided upon cast application but during the placing of this large patient in position of the table, the fracture became disimpacted and rotated. The doctor now should:
   A. Continue manipulation to regain reduction
   B. Prepare for open reduction
   C. Try various positions in traction
   D. Permit non-union to occur in the present position
   E. None of the above

332. At open reduction, the head fragment was entirely free in the joint with the ligamentum terest torn loose. Procedure should be:
   A. Fix head back in place with screws
   B. Maintain with a metal plate
   C. Use a sliding bone graft
   D. Remove the head and plan on a prosthetic replacement
   E. Remove the head and do arthroplasty
                                            Ref. 6 - p. 1819

CASE (Questions 333-336): A 60-year-old man complained of pain in the muscles of both shoulders for 3 months. He stated that he was also chronically weak and tired. Recently the muscle pains in the shoulders have become more severe. He had been a heavy smoker for many years but gave up smoking a month ago because he coughed up some blood. On examination, a faint erythematous macular rash was noted on the chest over the sternal area. His vital signs were normal. The deltoid muscles bilaterally were tender to touch and the skin was red and brawny. No appreciable wasting of musculature was noted. His deep tendon reflexes were hypoactive but sensory examination did not reveal any deficits. Physical examination of the lungs was negative as was the remainder of the physical examination.

333. The most probable diagnosis in this patient is:
   A. Polymyalgia rheumatica
   B. Dermatomyositis
   C. Trichinosis
   D. Syringomyelia of the cervical spinal cord
   E. Bilateral subachromial bursitis

334. Which one of the following tests or procedures would be most helpful in making a diagnosis?
   A. Temporal artery biopsy   D. Myelogram
   B. Deltoid muscle biopsy   E. X-rays of both shoulder
   C. Skin test for trichinosis   joints

335. The history of hemoptysis should alert the physician to the possibility of:
   A. Rheumatoid lung disease
   B. Bronchogenic carcinoma
   C. Congenital arteriovenous fistula in the lung
   D. Apical tuberculosis of the lung
   E. Eosinophilic pneumonia

336. Significant symptomatic relief is often possible with the use of:
   A. INH, PAS and streptomycin
   B. Hyperbaric oxygen
   C. Corticosteroids
   D. Intramuscular gold salts
   E. Injection of novocaine in the subachromial bursae
                                            Ref. 2 - p. 128

CASE (Questions 337-340): A healthy infant presents with sudden swelling of the lower part of the face. A fever of 102.8° F is found. The infant is very irritable and refuses feedings. The mother observes pallor and salivation. The child is examined by a physician and soft tissue swelling is found; the swelling is deep and firm and appears to be fixed to the mandible. There is no discoloration or increased local heat.

337. The most likely diagnosis is:
    A. Mumps
    B. Cervical adenitis
    C. Hypervitaminosis A
    D. Infantile cortical hyperostosis
    E. Syphilis

338. Which one of the following laboratory findings would be expected to be abnormal?
    A. Serum alkaline phosphatase
    B. BUN
    C. Serum electrolytes
    D. Sweat electrolytes
    E. Urine amino acids

339. The usual outcome of the disorder:
    A. Recovery in 3 days
    B. Recovery in several weeks or months
    C. Recovery in 6 months with osteomyelitis of sinuses
    D. Death in 7 days
    E. Death in 2 months

340. The child is best treated with:
    A. Penicillin
    B. 6-mercaptopurine
    C. Cortisone or hydrocortisone
    D. Hot soak, incision and drainage
    E. Amphotericin-B   Ref. 10 - p. 1741

CASE (Questions 341-344): A 40-year-old male underwent a cholecystectomy. He suffered a prolonged post-operative paralytic ileus and was maintained on intravenous fluids for seven days. On the seventh postoperative day, he was noted to be irrational and stuporous, with bizarre and rapidly changing neurologic signs. His serum sodium was found to be 112 mEq/L.

341. The most likely diagnosis here is:
    A. Inappropriate ADH secretion
    B. Dilutional hyponatremia
    C. Hypochloremic alkalosis
    D. Septicemia
    E. Meningitis
    Ref. 4 - p. 104

342. The most dangerous complication to expect next is:
    A. Metabolic alkalosis
    B. High fever
    C. Seizures
    D. Shock
    E. Renal failure
    Ref. 4 - p. 104

343. The most likely cause of this problem is:
    A. Elevated endogenous corticosteroids
    B. Elevated ADH
    C. Insufficient sodium administration
    D. Excessive administration of hypotonic solutions
    E. Inadequate potassium replacement
                                    Ref. 4 - p. 104

344. The best treatment in this setting is:
    A. Fluid restriction
    B. Hypertonic sodium intravenously
    C. Administration of both NaCl and KCl
    D. Hemodialysis
    E. "Loop" diuretics such as furosemide
                                    Ref. 4 - p. 104

CASE (Questions 345-348): A 40-year-old mother of five presents
with generalized weakness and dizziness of several month's duration,
together with difficulty in swallowing of one month's duration. Her
dietary intake has been extremely poor, and she also reports that
her menstrual flow has increased in volume for the past year.
Physical examination reveals a pale woman with abnormalities in the
appearance of her nails and mouth. Her peripheral blood smear
demonstrates hypochromic, microcytic red cells.

345. Which of the following is most probably increased in serum?
    A. Carotene   D. Calcium
    B. Vitamin B_{12} E. Glucose
    C. Iron binding capacity

346. Which of the following tests is most likely to be of diagnostic
    value?
    A. D-xylose excretion
    B. 131I triolein absorption
    C. Barium swallow of the esophagus
    D. 5-hydroxyindolacetic acid excretion
    E. Serum carotene concentration

347. The prognosis for the improvement of the dysphagia with proper
    treatment is:
    A. Poor   D. Good
    B. Fair   E. Excellent
    C. Unknown

348. Patients with this disorder probably have an increased incidence
    of:
    A. Achalasia   D. Hiatus hernia
    B. Carcinoma of the esophagus E. Scleroderma
    C. Peptic ulcer   Ref. 2 - p. 1179

CASE (Questions 349-352): A 45-year-old female suddenly complained of right lateral chest pain aggravated by cough and deep inspiration. She also coughed up some blood-tinged sputum. Examination of this afebrile female revealed marked splinting of the right hemithorax and a tachycardia of 110/min. There was acute tenderness, swelling and redness of the left calf. X-ray of the chest taken 3 days after the initial examination revealed a small right pleural effusion.

349. The most probable diagnosis is:
   A. Rupture of a subpleural bleb
   B. Acute pancreatitis
   C. Pulmonary tuberculosis with pleural effusion
   D. Pulmonary infarction with pleural effusion
   E. Early right lower lobe pneumonia

350. Confirmation of this diagnosis may be achieved by obtaining a:
   A. Timed vital capacity
   B. Phonocardiogram
   C. Pleural biopsy
   D. Serum amylase
   E. Pulmonary angiogram

351. The cardiac findings in this illness may include:
   A. Prominent pulsations in the second left intercostal space
   B. Accentuated pulmonary second sound
   C. Pleuropericardial friction rub
   D. Gallop rhythm
   E. All of the above

352. The management of this patient may include:
   A. Oxygen
   B. Anticoagulants
   C. Elastic stockings
   D. All of the above
   E. None of the above
   Ref. 2 - pp. 917-919

CASE (Questions 353-356): A 32-year-old man sustained a mid-shaft humeral fracture after very slight exertion. X-ray showed the fracture to be through a bone cyst and other films showed wide-spread bone cysts in other bones. The abdominal film showed a kidney stone.

353. The important diagnostic test is:
   A. Gastric juice for tumor cells
   B. Blood for acid phosphatase
   C. Spinal fluid colloidal gold
   D. Urine for calcium
   E. Blood for amylase
   Ref. 6 - p. 1478

354. The differential diagnosis includes all, except:
   A. Renal rickets
   B. Giant cell tumor of bone
   C. Hyperparathyroidism
   D. Kidney cancer with metastases
   E. Hypoparathyroidism
   Ref. 6 - p. 1488

355. If four parathyroid glands in this case are exposed at operation
     and no adenoma is found, the procedure of choice is to resect
     _____ glands:
     A. 1   D. 3-$\frac{1}{2}$
     B. 2   E. 4
     C. 3   Ref. 4 - p. 665

356. If bone involvement is extensive and surgical treatment of
     hyperparathyroidism is successful, the hypocalcemic tetany
     which immediately follows operation may be treated by:
     A. Parathyroid extract   D. Vitamin D
     B. Intravenous or oral calcium E. Any of the above
     C. Dihydrotachysterol   Ref. 4 - p. 666

     For each of the questions or incomplete statements below,
     one or more of the answers or completions given is correct.
     Answer according to the following key:

     A. If only 1, 2 and 3 are correct
     B. If only 1 and 3 are correct
     C. If only 2 and 4 are correct
     D. If only 4 is correct
     E. If all are correct

357. Functioning islet cell adenoma of the pancreas can be diagnosed
     by which of the following (Whipple's signs)?
     1. Attacks while fasting or fatigued
     2. Prompt relief after glucose administration
     3. Blood sugar level of less than 50 mgm/%
     4. Profuse sweating and palpitation
                                            Ref. 6 - p. 1275

358. The higher rate of mortality in emergency operation for in-
     carcerated inguinal hernia is due to:
     1. Bowel complications
     2. Anesthetic problems
     3. Concomitant disease
     4. Blood loss   Ref. 6 - p. 1351

359. Indications for adenoidectomy in a child include:
     1. Serous otitis media
     2. Chronic otitis media
     3. Chronic sinusitis
     4. Recurrent acute otitis media   Ref. 4 - p. 1221

360. Which of the following is apt to be the earliest postoperative
     evidence of common bile duct injury?
     1. Cholangitis
     2. Obstructive jaundice
     3. Bile peritonitis shock
     4. Excessive bile drainage from the wound
                                            Ref. 6 - p. 1232

ANSWER KEY

1. E	51. D	101. D	151. D	201. D
2. A	52. B	102. A	152. B	202. B
3. E	53. D	103. D	153. E	203. A
4. D	54. E	104. A	154. A	204. B
5. B	55. E	105. D	155. B	205. D
6. A	56. C	106. E	156. C	206. C
7. B	57. E	107. C	157. D	207. A
8. C	58. A	108. C	158. E	208. E
9. D	59. A	109. D	159. D	209. B
10. D	60. E	110. B	160. B	210. A
11. C	61. E	111. D	161. C	211. C
12. A	62. B	112. B	162. D	212. C
13. E	63. C	113. E	163. D	213. D
14. D	64. E	114. A	164. E	214. E
15. C	65. A	115. B	165. C	215. B
16. B	66. C	116. D	166. B	216. A
17. A	67. A	117. B	167. D	217. C
18. A	68. A	118. E	168. B	218. D
19. B	69. C	119. D	169. D	219. C
20. A	70. C	120. B	170. E	220. A
21. B	71. B	121. E	171. A	221. B
22. C	72. B	122. A	172. E	222. E
23. D	73. A	123. E	173. C	223. D
24. A	74. D	124. B	174. D	224. B
25. A	75. B	125. A	175. A	225. A
26. B	76. E	126. E	176. C	226. D
27. B	77. B	127. B	177. E	227. C
28. E	78. D	128. A	178. B	228. E
29. C	79. D	129. A	179. C	229. E
30. A	80. E	130. C	180. E	230. C
31. D	81. C	131. E	181. A	231. C
32. D	82. D	132. D	182. D	232. A
33. E	83. D	133. D	183. A	233. B
34. B	84. D	134. B	184. E	234. C
35. C	85. B	135. D	185. D	235. B
36. B	86. B	136. D	186. C	236. A
37. D	87. D	137. C	187. A	237. E
38. A	88. E	138. D	188. D	238. D
39. A	89. A	139. C	189. D	239. A
40. C	90. E	140. E	190. C	240. E
41. D	91. C	141. A	191. E	241. B
42. D	92. C	142. C	192. A	242. D
43. B	93. C	143. E	193. B	243. C
44. A	94. B	144. D	194. D	244. E
45. B	95. C	145. C	195. B	245. C
46. D	96. C	146. D	196. C	246. B
47. B	97. D	147. B	197. A	247. A
48. D	98. A	148. D	198. D	248. D
49. B	99. D	149. A	199. C	249. B
50. B	100. D	150. D	200. E	250. E

ANSWER KEY

251. D	301. B	351. E
252. A	302. A	352. D
253. C	303. B	353. D
254. A	304. A	354. E
255. B	305. B	355. D
256. B	306. B	356. E
257. B	307. C	357. A
258. A	308. C	358. B
259. A	309. C	359. E
260. D	310. C	360. D
261. A	311. B	
262. B	312. D	
263. D	313. E	
264. C	314. E	
265. B	315. A	
266. B	316. B	
267. B	317. B	
268. C	318. C	
269. B	319. C	
270. A	320. D	
271. C	321. A	
272. C	322. D	
273. D	323. E	
274. A	324. C	
275. B	325. C	
276. C	326. C	
277. D	327. C	
278. B	328. C	
279. C	329. A	
280. C	330. E	
281. A	331. B	
282. C	332. D	
283. B	333. B	
284. B	334. B	
285. B	335. B	
286. A	336. C	
287. B	337. D	
288. C	338. A	
289. B	339. B	
290. D	340. C	
291. A	341. B	
292. C	342. C	
293. A	343. D	
294. C	344. B	
295. B	345. C	
296. B	346. C	
297. C	347. E	
298. A	348. B	
299. A	349. D	
300. C	350. E	

SECOND EXAMINATION

For each of the following multiple choice questions, select the one most appropriate answer:

1. At 15 months a child would be expected to do all of the following, except:
   A. Walk alone and crawl up stairs
   B. Handle a spoon well
   C. Make a tower of 2 cubes;insert a pellet into a bottle
   D. Indicate desires by pointing
   E. Follow simple commands   Ref. 11 - p. 50

2. Adequate treatment of benign prostatic hypertrophy is by:
   A. Regimen of massage   D. Resection
   B. Hormone therapy   E. Suprapubic drainage
   C. Antibiotics   Ref. 4 - p. 1546

3. Acute mastitis most commonly occurs early in:
   A. The normal menstrual cycle   D. Pregnancy
   B. Puberty   E. Menopause
   C. Lactation   Ref. 4 - p. 577

4. Current thought is that the postgastrectomy "dumping" syndrome is due to:
   A. Serotonin release
   B. "Dumping" of hypertonic material into the jejunum
   C. Hypoglycemia
   D. Sudden hypovolemia
   E. Small gastric pouch   Ref. 6 - p. 1065

5. Uremic manifestations in patients with acute renal failure:
   A. Tend to be very severe
   B. Are usually minimal
   C. Are less than those in patients with chronic renal failure
   D. Never include gastrointestinal effects
   E. Usually spare the central nervous system
                                   Ref. 2 - p. 1111

6. During thyroidectomy, damage to the superior laryngeal nerve causes:
   A. No effect
   B. Loss of timbre and resonance of the voice
   C. Hoarseness
   D. Paralysis of the vocal cords
   E. Loss of speech   Ref. 4 - p. 627

7. Disorders of coagulation usually have:
   A. Normal platelet counts   D. All of the above
   B. Normal tourniquet test   E. None of the above
   C. Normal bleeding time   Ref. 1 - p. 306

8. When renal injury is suspected, intravenous pyelogram should be done:
   A. Only if there is hematuria   D. Electively in most cases
   B. Only if there is oliguria   E. Immediately in most cases
   C. Only if there is anuria   Ref. 4 - p. 386

9. Venous drainage of the upper part of the uterus and placental site is via the:
   A. Uterine   D. Ovarian
   B. Hypogastric   E. Superior vesicle
   C. Internal iliac   Ref. 7 - p. 978

10. Laboratory data in von Willebrand's disease include:
    A. Normal partial thromboplastin time
    B. Normal prothrombin time
    C. Decreased platelets
    D. All of the above
    E. None of the above   Ref. 1 - p. 308

11. When an extremity has been ischemic for more than ____ hours, and flow is restored, fasciotomy should be done.
    A. 2 hours   D. Rarely, if ever
    B. 4 hours   E. In all cases
    C. 6 hours   Ref. 4 - p. 392

12. Diagnostic findings in chronic constrictive pericarditis do not include:
    A. Enlarged liver with ascites
    B. Absence of murmurs or abnormal sounds
    C. Enlarged heart
    D. Decreased or absent cardiac impulse
    E. Distended peripheral veins and heart failure
                                          Ref. 6 - p. 802

13. Which is not true regarding enchondroma?
    A. Usually found in interior of small bones of hands and feet
    B. Lesion resembles hyaline cartilage
    C. Fusiform swelling of bone may result
    D. Surrounding cortex is thickened
    E. Pathologic fracture is frequent   Ref. 4 - p. 1387

14. The safest way to deliver a persistent occiput posterior:
    A. Manual rotation
    B. Scanzoni maneuver
    C. Rotation and delivery with Kielland forceps
    D. C-section
    E. Deliver as posterior with forceps   Ref. 7 - p. 853

15. The normal myeloid/erythroid (M/E) ratio is approximately:
    A. 1:1   D. 1:3
    B. 4:1   E. None of the above
    C. 1:4   Ref. 1 - p. 298

16. All of the following are characteristic of sensorineural hearing loss, <u>except</u>:
    A. High frequencies tend to be more affected than low tones
    B. Sounds appear distorted
    C. Sound discrimination is impaired
    D. Generally result in greater handicap to communication than do conductive losses
    E. Respond well to surgical therapy   Ref. 11 - pp. 118-119

17. The most important step in the treatment of a badly infected episiotomy is:
    A. Hot sitz baths   D. Drainage
    B. Antibiotics   E. Relief of pain by narcotics
    C. Securing cultures of wounds   Ref. 7 - p. 977

18. In Gilbert's syndrome, there is:
    A. Increased frequency of peptic ulcer
    B. Unconjugated hyperbilirubinemia
    C. Conjugated bilirubinemia
    D. Increased transferase activity
    E. Frequent attacks of biliary colic   Ref. 2 - p. 1335

19. Regarding manipulation and cast treatment of talipes equinovarus:
    A. Forefoot adduction is corrected first
    B. Heel eversion is corrected first
    C. Dorsiflexion of the foot is corrected first
    D. All are corrected by the first cast application
    E. Cast change is made every six weeks
                                     Ref. 6 - p. 1733

20. The most common cause of acute cervicitis is:
    A. E. coli   D. Streptococcus
    B. Hemophilis vaginalis   E. Staphylococcus
    C. Gonorrhea   Ref. 8 - pp. 395-398

21. Diagnosis of adrenal insufficiency in the absence of crises depends upon:
    A. Reduction in plasma 17-hydroxycorticoids and failure to rise after corticotropin
    B. Lack of increase in urinary excretion of 17-keto and 11-hydroxy steroids after corticotropin
    C. Lack of adequate urine volume increase after water load
    D. Increase in Na/K ratio above 2.0 in saliva
    E. Any of the above   Ref. 4 - p. 689

22. Absence of one umbilical artery occurs in ____ of single pregnancies:
    A. 0.5%   D. 5%
    B. 1%   E. 7%
    C. 3%   Ref. 7 - pp. 598-599

23. Medullary carcinoma of the thyroid is associated with all of the
    following, except:
    A. Calcitonin
    B. Serotonin
    C. Prostaglandins
    D. Multiple endocrine adenomatosis
    E. Better prognosis than papillary carcinoma

    Ref. 4 - p. 639

24. The best surgical treatment for mild hallux valgus without osteo-
    arthritis is:
    A. Excision of bursa, exostosis and prominent medial aspect of
       metatarsal head
    B. Excision of bursa, exostosis and proximal half of proximal
       phalanx
    C. Excision of bursa, exostosis and entire metatarsal head
    D. Arthrodesis of metatarso-phalangeal joint
    E. Amputation of great toe   Ref. 6 - p. 1868

25. Single pigmented nevi on the hand may be premalignant. They
    should be:
    A. Excised   D. Cauterized
    B. Irradiated   E. Left alone
    C. Fulgurated   Ref. 4 - p. 1450

26. Call-exner bodies are associated with:
    A. Arrhenoblastomas   D. Granulosa cell tumors
    B. Brenner tumors   E. Dysgerminomas
    C. Hilar cell tumors   Ref. 8 - p. 515

27. Jaundice is usually detected clinically in the sclerae when the
    serum concentration of bilirubin is greater than:
    A. 1-2 mg per 100 ml   D. 3-5 mg per 100 ml
    B. 0.5-1 mg per 100 ml   E. Greater than 5 mg per
    C. 2-3 mg per 100 ml   100 ml
                                Ref. 2 - p. 1324

28. Striking enlargement of the chorionic villi is commonly seen
    in:
    A. Erythroblastosis   D. Renal disease
    B. Toxemia of pregnancy E. Syphilis
    C. Diabetes   Ref. 7 - p. 592

29. Mycotic vulvitis is frequently associated with:
    A. Lymphomas   D. Leukemia
    B. Tuberculosis   E. Allergies
    C. Diabetes   Ref. 8 - p. 183

30. Incriminated factors in bladder tumor causation include:
    A. Aniline dye   D. Chronic irritation
    B. Bilharziasis   E. All of the above
    C. Body metabolites   Ref. 6 - p. 1573

31. In Huntington's chorea, degenerative changes often extensively
    involve the:
    A. Pons   D. Red nucleus
    B. Caudate nucleus   E. Substantia nigra
    C. Cerebellum   Ref. 2 - p. 642

32. Down syndrome (21-trisomy) is not associated with:
    A. Abnormal development of skull and characteristic facies
    B. Tongue protrusion as a result of small oral cavity
    C. Generalized hypertonia during infancy
    D. Cardiac anomalies often involving atrio-ventricular structure
    E. Mental deficiency usually of moderate to severe range
                                    Ref. 11 - pp. 134-136

33. The drug most often effective in treating the Hamman-Rich
    syndrome is:
    A. Adrenal steroids   D. PAS
    B. Vitamin B_{12} E. Sulfonamides
    C. INH   Ref. 2 - p. 849

34. Which of the following rule out radical mastectomy for breast
    cancer?
    A. Proven distant metastasis
    B. Skin ulceration
    C. Fixation of lesion to chest wall
    D. Fixation of enlarged axillary nodes
    E. All of the above   Ref. 6 - p. 561

35. In hemochromatosis increased infiltration of the liver with
    _____ occurs:
    A. Fat   D. Copper
    B. Amyloid   E. Zinc
    C. Iron   Ref. 2 - p. 1467

36. Huntington's chorea is recognized by the triad of familial in-
    cidence, choreiform movements, and:
    A. Dementia   D. Convulsions
    B. Oculogyric crises   E. Aphasia
    C. Nystagmus   Ref. 2 - p. 642

37. A suitable mechanism for attaining more nerve length in the
    suture of peripheral nerves is:
    A. Gentle traction on nerve ends
    B. Mobilization of distal and proximal segments
    C. Joint flexion and extremity positioning
    D. Nerve transposition
    E. Any of the above   Ref. 4 - p. 1308

38. Athetosis is most often found in association with:
    A. Multiple sclerosis   D. Huntington's chorea
    B. Parkinson's disease   E. Lipidoses
    C. Cerebral palsy   Ref. 2 - p. 643

39. If a thyroid nodule is ___ to I^{131} and ___ to Se ^{75}, it has a
    50% chance of being malignant.
    A. "Cold", "hot"   D. "Hot", "hot"
    B. "Cold", "cold"   E. Se^{75} is not used in thyroid
    C. "Hot", "cold"   scanning
                                         Ref. 4 - p. 644

40. In the spontaneous hyperplasia of hyperthyroidism, administra-
    tion of iodine:
    A. Causes involution of the thyroid gland
    B. Returns the gland to normal
    C. Has no effect on the anterior pituitary
    D. Increases secretion of TSH
    E. Has a secretory-stimulating effect on the thyroid
                                         Ref. 4 - p. 624

41. Hemiballism may be produced by lesions of the:
    A. Cerebral cortex   D. Corpus Luysii
    B. Cerebellar cortex   E. Caudate nucleus
    C. Substantia nigra   Ref. 2 - p. 645

42. The typical patient with ureteral calculus presents with which
    principal complaint?
    A. Nocturia   D. Hematuria
    B. Palpable mass   E. Urgency and incontinence
    C. Renal colic   Ref. 6 - p. 1562

43. The Budd-Chiari syndrome is due to occlusion of the:
    A. Portal veins   D. Pancreatic veins
    B. Hepatic veins   E. Mesenteric veins
    C. Splenic veins   Ref. 2 - p. 1346

44. During infancy, the caloric requirement is:
    A. 50 calories/Kg.   D. 150 calories/Kg.
    B. 70 calories/Kg.   E. 175 calories/Kg.
    C. 110 calories/Kg.   Ref. 11 - p. 175

45. The incidence of hepatoma is increased to the greatest extent
    in patients with:
    A. Laennec's cirrhosis   D. Portal hypertension
    B. Hypoglycemia   E. Cholestatic jaundice
    C. Hemochromatosis   Ref. 2 - p. 1352

46. Examination of the peripheral blood smear of a splenectomized
    patient in the postoperative period may reveal the presence of:
    A. Neutrophilia   D. Target cells
    B. Thrombocytosis   E. All of the above
    C. Howell-Jolly bodies   Ref. 1 - p. 311

47. Delayed clamping of the cord:
    A. Is a benefit in the isoimmunized infant
    B. Is a benefit to the premature infant
    C. May give the infant as much as 100 ml of blood
    D. Increases risk of circulatory failure due to hypervolemia
    E. May be of value in preventing respiratory distress syndrome
                                            Ref. 7 - p. 415

48. The most common site of endometriosis is:
    A. Uterosacral ligaments   D. Umbilicus
    B. Rectovaginal septum   E. Laparotomy scars
    C. Round ligaments   Ref. 8 - p. 542

49. _____ is the major estrogen produced during pregnancy.
    A. Ethinyl estradiol   D. Estrone
    B. Estradiol   E. Ethisterone
    C. Estriol   Ref. 7 - pp. 177-184

50. The decidua capsularis is:
    A. That portion on which the ovum rests
    B. That portion of decidua vera which covers the ovum
    C. Lines the major portion of the uterus
    D. Adheres to opposing wall of uterus with growth of ovum
    E. The thickest at the fourth month of pregnancy
                                            Ref. 7 - p. 146

51. In figuring electrolyte requirement for the first 24 hours after
    serious thermal injury, which of the following is correct?
    A. Use lactated Ringer's solution in saline with caution
    B. Allow for salt in plasma and decrease accordingly
    C. 0.5 ml/Kg body wt/% body surface burn
    D. 1.5 ml/Kg body wt/% body surface burn
    E. 1.0 ml/Kg body wt/% body surface burn
                                            Ref. 6 - p. 261

52. Parathyroid carcinoma presents as:
    A. Primary hyperparathyroidism D. Hoarseness of the voice
    B. A mass in the neck   E. Hypothyroidism
    C. Asymptomatic   Ref. 4 - p. 659

53. A _____ type of placenta is found in man:
    A. Epitheliochorial
    B. Syndesmochorial
    C. Endotheliochorial
    D. Hemochorial   Ref. 7 - p. 186

54. Kwashiorkor (protein malnutrition) is characterized by:
    A. Early development of edema
    B. Infection constitutes the most important added stress
    C. Dermatitis is common
    D. All of the above
    E. None of the above   Ref. 11 - pp. 183-186

55. The coagulation factor necessary for both the partial thrombo-
    plastin time and the prothrombin time determinations is:
    A. XII   D. VIII
    B. X   E. IX
    C. VII   Ref. 1 - p. 306

56. Most deaths involving placenta previa result from:
    A. Infection   D. Thrombophlebitis
    B. Toxemia   E. Traumatic rupture of uterus
    C. Hemorrhage   Ref. 7 - p. 613

57. Carcinoma which has metastasized to lymph nodes produces
    nodes which are:
    A. Soft and matted   D. Soft and fluctuant
    B. Fluctuant   E. Rubbery
    C. Very hard   Ref. 1 - p. 310

58. The Folds of Hoboken are found in:
    A. New Jersey   D. The umbilical cord
    B. The placenta   E. The ductus venosus
    C. The amnion   Ref. 7 - p. 173

59. Pathological conditions that show autosomal recessive inheri-
    tance include all of the following, except:
    A. Progressive muscular dystrophy (Duchenne type)
    B. Adrenogenital syndrome
    C. Thalassemia major
    D. Cystic fibrosis
    E. Gargoylism   Ref. 11 - p. 294

60. The main hazard in operation for mediastinal pheochromocytoma
    is:
    A. Excessive release of catecholamines
    B. Failure to remove all of the tumor
    C. Damage to the thoracic duct
    D. Damage to the posterior nerve roots
    E. Uncontrollable hemorrhage   Ref. 6 - p. 669

61. Which one of the following is increased in incidence in patients
    with obstructive pulmonary emphysema?
    A. Intestinal polyposis   D. Insulinoma
    B. Colonic diverticulae   E. Regional ileitis
    C. Peptic ulcer   Ref. 1 - p. 1434

62. Which one of the following maternal medications has been as-
    sociated with abortion and thrombocytopenia:
    A. Preludin   D. Tetracycline
    B. Propylthiouracil   E. Thalidomide
    C. Quinine   Ref. 11 - p. 324

63. In Erb-Duchenne paralysis, the newborn:
    A. Loses the power to abduct the arm from the shoulder
    B. Cannot rotate the arm externally
    C. Cannot supinate the forearm
    D. All of the above
    E. None of the above   Ref. 11 - p. 355

64. The longest diameter of the fetal skull is:
    A. Bitemporal   D. Biparietal
    B. Suboccipitalbregmatic   E. Occipitofrontal
    C. Occipitomental   Ref. 7 - pp. 205,868

65. In advanced prostatic cancer:
    A. Sciatic pain is a rare occurrence
    B. Serum acid and alkaline phosphatase are elevated only with
       metastases
    C. Frequency and nocturia are the usual early symptoms
    D. Isolated osteolytic metastases are common
    E. Pulmonary metastases are large and frequent
                                 Ref. 6 - p. 1578

66. Marked lymphadenopathy is noted commonly in all of the follow-
    ing except:
    A. Chronic lymphocytic leukemia D. Chronic myelogenous leu-
    B. Hodgkin's disease   kemia
    C. Lymphosarcoma   E. None of the above
                                      Ref. 1 - p. 313

67. After peripheral nerve suture, estimated functional growth is
    about _____ inches per month.
    A. 0.5   D. 3
    B. 1   E. 4
    C. 2   Ref. 6 - p. 1644

68. Demargination may be the mechanism leading to neutrophilia in:
    A. Epinephrine injections   D. None of the above
    B. Delirium tremens   E. All of the above
    C. Paroxysmal tachycardia   Ref. 1 - p. 316

69. The approach to adrenalectomy with the least morbidity is:
    A. Abdominal, intraperitoneal
    B. Abdominal, extraperitoneal
    C. Thoracoabdominal
    D. Thoracotomy and division of diaphragm
    E. Posterior   Ref. 4 - p. 687

70. Patients with caustic burns of the esophagus are best treated with:
    A. Nasogastric tube and tube feedings
    B. Intravenous hyperalimentation
    C. Corticosteroids, antibiotics and nothing by mouth
    D. Corticosteroids, antibiotics and early feedings
    E. Corticosteroids, antibiotics and late (10 days) feedings
                                  Ref. 4 - p. 758

71. Urgent operation in tetralogy of Fallot is to:
    A. Prevent death
    B. Decrease anoxia
    C. Prevent hemiplegia
    D. Decrease cyanosis
    E. All of the above
    Ref. 6 - p. 722

72. The acute renal failure due to acute tubular necrosis differs from
    the acute renal failure due to volume depletion in that the former
    is usually characterized by:
    A. Low BUN
    B. Low plasma creatinine
    C. Decreased sodium excretion
    D. Increased excretion of water in relation to the glomerular
       filtration rate
    E. Decreased excretion of water in relation to the glomerular
       filtration rate
    Ref. 2 - p. 1110

73. Contraindication to operation for mitral stenosis is:
    A. Episode of cerebral embolization
    B. Advanced disease
    C. Severe pulmonary hypertension
    D. Calcified valve
    E. None of the above
    Ref. 6 - p. 766

74. Which type of brain damage is seen in cyanotic heart disease
    children:
    A. Periodic episodes of unconsciousness
    B. Brain abscess
    C. Localized infarct
    D. Paradoxical embolism
    E. All of the above
    Ref. 6 - p. 681

75. In a normal pregnancy the peak of chorionic gonadotropin is
    found at:
    A. 100-120 days
    B. 30-40 days
    C. 50-80 days
    D. 200-210 days
    E. Term
    Ref. 8 - pp. 50-54

76. Which one of the following findings is commonly seen in patients
    with right-to-left shunt?
    A. Cyanosis
    B. Clubbing of the fingers and toes
    C. Secondary polycythemia
    D. All of the above
    E. None of the above
    Ref. 1 - p. 1157

77. Hydramnios is associated with:
    A. Anencephaly
    B. Malformation of gastrointestinal tract
    C. Erythroblastosis
    D. None
    E. All
    Ref. 7 - pp. 599-600

78. An increased percentage of plasma cells in the marrow may be noted in:
    A. Chronic liver disease   D. All of the above
    B. Aplastic anemia   E. None of the above
    C. Multiple myeloma   Ref. 1 - p. 322

79. Which type of pulmonary neoplasm is most often associated with cigarette smoking?
    A. Adenocarcinoma   D. Lymphoma
    B. Squamous cell carcinoma   E. All of the above
    C. Alveolar cell carcinoma   Ref. 1 - p. 1323

80. All of the following statements concerning berry aneurysms are true except:
    A. They are found in association with polycystic kidneys
    B. They are found in association with aortic coarctation
    C. Most arise in the circle of Willis
    D. A very high familial incidence is noted
    E. They probably arise from congenital defects
                                      Ref. 2 - p. 663

81. Angiokeratoma corporis diffusum universale (Fabry's disease) is due to an intracellular accumulation of:
    A. Ceramide trihexoside   D. Sphingomyelin
    B. Cholesterol esters   E. Mucopolysaccharides
    C. Tryptophan   Ref. 11 - pp. 1540-1541

82. The solid mass of cells early in ovum development is called:
    A. Blastocyst   D. Morula
    B. Blastomere   E. None of the above
    C. Gastrula   Ref. 7 - p. 128

83. Oxytocin:
    A. Induces vigorous sustained uterine contraction
    B. Comes from the anterior pituitary
    C. Possesses no antidiuretic activity
    D. Must be used with care because of its vasopressor activity
    E. Acts on myoepithelial cells of mammary glands
                                      Ref. 7 - p. 419

84. Subarachnoid hemorrhage occurs most commonly as a result of:
    A. Trauma
    B. Rupture of a berry aneurysm
    C. Rupture of a fusiform aneurysm
    D. Rupture of a mycotic aneurysm
    E. Rupture of an A-V anomaly   Ref. 2 - p. 664

85. A primigravida at term is found to have a breech presentation during the first stage of labor. The next step would be:
    A. Attempt external version
    B. C-section
    C. Rupture the membranes
    D. X-ray studies of fetus and pelvis
    E. Apply an abdominal binder
    Ref. 7 - p. 862

86. Generalized peritonitis secondary to puerperal endometritis is best treated by:
    A. Hysterectomy
    B. Laparotomy and drainage of abdomen
    C. Antibiotics, gastrointestinal suction and fluids
    D. Antibiotics and intrauterine douches
    E. Antibiotics and D & C   Ref. 7 - pp. 984-985

87. Adequate immobilization is essential from the time of fracture until bone regeneration is solid in order to prevent:
    A. Damage to adjacent nerves and vessels
    B. Angulation and shortening
    C. Mal or nonunion
    D. Pain
    E. All of the above   Ref. 4 - p. 1329

88. Which of the following factors is not required for the process of blood coagulation via the intrinsic pathway?
    A. VII
    B. VIII
    C. IX
    D. XI
    E. XII
    Ref. 1 - p. 306

89. Acute intermittent porphyria is characterized by:
    A. Transmission as an autosomal recessive
    B. Clinical onset during early childhood and infancy
    C. Acute visceral and neurological attacks
    D. Presence of cutaneous lesions
    E. All of the above   Ref. 11 - p. 470

90. The most important diagnostic sign of substernal goiter is:
    A. Deviation of the trachea on X-ray film
    B. Dilatation of neck veins
    C. Dyspnea and orthopnea
    D. Choking and coughing in sleep
    E. Fullness in suprasternal notch   Ref. 6 - p. 664

91. Of the following hormones, which is not secreted by the anterior pituitary lobe?
    A. Growth hormone (GH)
    B. Thyroid stimulating hormone (TSH)
    C. Follicle stimulating hormone (FSH)
    D. Melanocyte stimulating hormone (MSH)
    E. Adrenocorticotropic hormone (ACTH)
    Ref. 6 - p. 1365

92. Clinical manifestations of asthma include all of the following,
   except:
   A. Asthmatic paroxysm associated with prolongation of expira-
   tion
   B. Heart rate increased
   C. Restlessness and sweating
   D. Sputum is watery and copious
   E. Chest usually hyperresonant   Ref. 11 - p. 505

93. Laboratory findings associated with juvenile rheumatoid arthri-
   tis:
   A. Sedimentation rate usually elevated
   B. Anemia is common
   C. White blood cell count often elevated
   D. All of the above
   E. None of the above   Ref. 11 - p. 527

94. ____% of patients with perforated peptic ulcers show free air
   under the diaphragm on upright chest X-ray.
   A. 25%   D. 90%
   B. 50%   E. Almost 100%
   C. 75%   Ref. 4 - p. 835

95. The most frequent complication of Curling's ulcer in severe
   burns is:
   A. Hemorrhage   D. Paralytic ileus
   B. Perforation   E. Obstruction
   C. Pain   Ref. 6 - p. 992

96. The treatment of Zollinger-Ellison syndrome is:
   A. Vagotomy and pyloroplasty D. Total gastrectomy
   B. Vagotomy and antrectomy   E. Resection of the pancreatic
   C. Subtotal gastrectomy   tumor
                                 Ref. 4 - p. 841

97. The half-life of bromide in the blood is approximately:
   A. 20 minutes   D. 12 days
   B. 2-4 hours   E. 3 months
   C. 24-48 hours   Ref. 2 - p. 592

98. Berry aneurysm rupture is associated with ____% mortality
   for each major attack:
   A. 5%   D. 75%
   B. 25%   E. 95%
   C. 45%   Ref. 2 - p. 667

99. ____% of patients with Crohn's disease are permanently cured
   by a single resection.
   A. Less than 10%   D. 75%
   B. 25%   E. 90%
   C. 50%   Ref. 4 - p. 900

100. _____ are associated with gestational trophoblastic disease.
      A. Mesotheliomas   D. Theca lutein cysts
      B. Benign cystic teratomas   E. All of the above
      C. Serous cystadenoma   Ref. 8 - pp. 587, 594

101. When lumbar puncture reveals high CSF pressure:
      A. Enough fluid should be removed to lower the pressure
      B. Queckenstedt's test should always be performed
      C. The pressure should always be measured after jugular com-
         pression
      D. All of the above
      E. None of the above   Ref. 2 - p. 670

102. ____ % of all colonic carcinomas are within reach of the sig-
      moidoscope.
      A. 10%   D. 75%
      B. 25%   E. 90%
      C. 50%   Ref. 4 - p. 947

103. The Schultz-Charlton test, Pastia's lines, and brawny desqua-
      mation are of diagnostic value in:
      A. Diphtheria   D. Smallpox
      B. Scarlet fever   E. German measles
      C. Measles   Ref. 11 - pp. 570-571

104. Squamous cell skin cancer:
      A. Is most common in dark-haired persons
      B. Metastasizes by blood stream
      C. Most prevalent in skin areas exposed to actinic rays
      D. Upper lip is the commonest site
      E. More responsive to irradiation than basal cell type
                                       Ref. 4 - p. 1444

105. In older children with severe cyanotic heart disease, which of
      the following is seen rarely or not at all?
      A. Increased bronchial circulation
      B. Hemoptysis
      C. Epistaxis
      D. Defects in blood coagulability
      E. Mediastinal varicosities   Ref. 6 - p. 681

106. The procedure of choice for obstructing stricture of the rectum
      secondary to lymphogranuloma venereum is:
      A. Temporary colostomy and corticosteroids
      B. Temporary colostomy and radiation
      C. Forceful dilatation
      D. Abdominoperineal resection
      E. Local fulguration   Ref. 4 - p. 960

107. The drug of choice in treating an infection of brucellosis of
average severity is:
A. Penicillin   D. Amphotericin B
B. Sulfonamide   E. Tetracycline
C. Chloramphenicol   Ref. 11 - p. 612

108. The body of a normal adult contains approximately _____ gms
of iron:
A. 10-15   D. 2-6
B. 0. 5-1   E. 25-35
C. 100-120   Ref. 1 - p. 1581

109. Which one of the following statements regarding Klebsiella
pneumonia is true?
A. It is more common in alcoholics
B. Red currant jelly sputum is often characteristic
C. Bulging fissures are commonly seen on an X-ray of chest
D. Penicillin is usually ineffective in the treatment
E. All of the above   Ref. 2 - p. 287

110. Neurological complications are more common with:
A. Measles   D. Roseola
B. Chickenpox   E. Fifth disease
C. German measles   Ref. 11 - p. 655

111. The gametogenesis, failure of a pair of chromosomes to sep-
arate during meiotic division, is referred to as:
A. Translocation   D. Dyskariosis
B. Nondisjunction   E. Conjointism
C. Inversion   Ref. 7 - p. 124

112. The cardiac arrest or ventricular fibrillation secondary to
coronary thrombosis and myocardial infarction often does not
respond to:
A. Electroshock
B. Mouth-to-mouth resuscitation
C. Cardiac massage
D. Drug administration
E. Any of the above   Ref. 6 - p. 759

113. Erythema infectiosum:
A. Requires a 7 day isolation period
B. Is usually first recognized with the appearance of a rash
C. Is usually complicated by otitis media
D. Is characterized by leukopenia and proteinuria
E. Is associated with spiking fevers
                Ref. 11 - pp. 663-664

114. Palatopharyngeal incompetence is characterized by all of the
following, except:
A. Hypernasal speech defect
B. Flaring of nares during speech

C. Inability to whistle or blow out a candle
D. Loss of liquid through nose when drinking with the head down
E. Otitis media and hearing loss

Ref. 11 - pp. 797-798

115. Severe hemolytic anemia, hyperlipemia and alcoholic hepatitis is known as:
A. Budd-Chiari syndrome
B. Gardner's syndrome
C. Peutz-Jeghers syndrome
D. Cruveilhier-Baumgarten syndrome
E. Zieve's syndrome

Ref. 2 - p. 1330

116. Villous adenomas of the rectum, if grossly benign, should be resected:
A. By colotomy and polypectomy
B. By segmental resection
C. Through the sigmoidoscope
D. Through the sigmoidoscope after radiation
E. By abdominoperineal resection   Ref. 4 - p. 964

117. The most common predisposing factor in pseudomembranous enterocolitis is:
A. Intestinal obstruction
B. Peritonitis
C. Oral antibiotic bowel preparation
D. Cortisone therapy
E. Hypovolemic shock   Ref. 6 - p. 1119

118. Carcinoma of the rectum less than 8 cm from the anus should be resected by:
A. Abdominoperineal resection
B. Anterior resection and primary anastomosis
C. Anterior resection and Hartmann colostomy
D. Fulguration
E. Any of the above combined with radiation

Ref. 4 - p. 970

119. CSF examination in acute bacterial meningitis usually reveals:
A. Predominant increase of lymphocytes
B. Normal CSF pressure
C. Protein usually 50-100
D. All of the above
E. None of the above   Ref. 2 - p. 670

120. Melena, hematemesis, and epigastric pain are usually associated with:
A. Peptic ulcer
B. Meckel's diverticulum
C. Anal fissure
D. Intestinal duplication
E. Volvulus

Ref. 11 - p. 833

121. The procedure which is of greatest value in making a positive
diagnosis of tuberculous peritonitis is:
   A. Tuberculin skin test
   B. Upper gastrointestinal contrast study
   C. Culture of peritoneal fluid
   D. Peritoneal biopsy
   E. Plain X-ray film of the abdomen
   Ref. 2 - p. 407

122. Brain abscess may be a complication of:
   A. Bronchiectasis   D. All of the above
   B. Lung abscess   E. None of the above
   C. Middle ear infection   Ref. 2 - p. 672

123. Which is false in regard to hypovolemic shock?
   A. Glucocorticoids are helpful in producing vasodilatation
   B. Combination of alpha-blocking and beta-stimulating drugs
      is beneficial
   C. Volume replacement usually is curative alone
   D. Vasoconstrictor drugs improve tissue perfusion
   E. Beta-stimulating drugs increase cardiac output if venous
      return is adequate   Ref. 6 - p. 134

124. Shoulder dystocia with large infants:
   A. Can be prevented by restricting mothers diet
   B. Frequently necessitates cleidotomy
   C. Often occurs in diabetic mothers
   D. Is best treated by C-section
   E. Is usually seen in contracted pelves
   Ref. 7 - pp. 881-882

125. If an undescended testis has too short a pedicle to permit
placement in the scrotum, one should:
   A. Leave it in the abdomen   D. Free-graft it in the thigh
   B. Excise it   E. Put it at the external ring
   C. Give hormone therapy   Ref. 4 - p. 1563

126. The suture uniting the two parietal bones to the occipital bone
in the fetal skull is:
   A. Coronal   D. Sagittal
   B. Lambdoid   E. Temporal
   C. Frontal   Ref. 7 - p. 204

127. Acute bacterial endocarditis may lead to:
   A. Brain abscess   D. All of the above
   B. Purulent meningitis   E. None of the above
   C. Embolic cerebral infarction   Ref. 2 - p. 677

128. In the Dukes classification of colonic carcinoma, a lesion classified as B_1:
    A. Is confined to the mucosa
    B. Extends to the muscularis mucosa, nodes negative
    C. Extends through the muscularis mucosa, nodes negative
    D. Extends through all coats of the bowel, nodes negative
    E. None of the above   Ref. 4 - p. 972

129. In toxic megacolon associated with ulcerative colitis, the treatment of choice is:
    A. Loop ileostomy and no resection
    B. Cecostomy and no resection
    C. Subtotal or total colectomy and ileostomy
    D. Antibiotics and corticosteroids and no surgery
    E. Antibiotics and corticosteroids and cecostomy
         Ref. 4 - p. 977

130. Transverse myelitis usually affects:
    A. Cervical and thoracic segments
    B. Thoracic and lumbar segments
    C. Lumbar and sacral segments
    D. Lumbar segments alone
    E. None of the above   Ref. 2 - p. 678

131. The most frequent early manifestation of pulmonary emboli in most patients is usually:
    A. Dyspnea
    B. Cyanosis
    C. Hemoptysis
    D. Pleuritic chest pain
    E. Leg edema
         Ref. 2 - p. 918

132. Diffuse pulmonary interstitial infiltration in a patient with diabetes insipidus and osteolytic bone lesions is most suggestive of:
    A. Systemic lupus erythematosus
    B. Hemochromatosis
    C. Goodpasture's syndrome
    D. Hand-Schüller-Christian disease
    E. Pulmonary alveolar microlithiasis
         Ref. 2 - p. 1529

133. The major laboratory abnormality found in Congenital Adrenal Hyperplasia is:
    A. Increased FSH
    B. Increased 17-ketosteroids
    C. Increased cortisol
    D. Decreased ACTH
    E. Increased 17-hydroxyprogesterone
         Ref. 8 - p. 670

134. A test useful for demonstrating that a patient is receiving drugs of the opiate type is the:
    A. Tensilon test
    B. Nalorphine test
    C. Secretin test
    D. Perchlorate test
    E. None of the above
         Ref. 2 - p. 603

135. The most common lesion of the placenta is:
    A. Infarct   D. Calcification
    B. Cyst   E. Inflammation
    C. Angioma   Ref. 7 - pp. 590-592

136. The drug of choice in the treatment of infections due to bacte-
    roides is usually:
    A. Streptomycin   D. Tetracycline
    B. Neomycin   E. None of the above
    C. Dapsone   Ref. 1 - p. 802

137. The commonest causative organism in osteomyelitis is:
    A. Streptococcus   D. Syphilis spirochete
    B. Staphylococcus   E. Pseudomonas
    C. Tubercle bacillus   Ref. 4 - p. 1383

138. Atresia is most common in the:
    A. Stomach   D. Ileum
    B. Duodenum   E. Colon
    C. Jejunum   Ref. 11 - p. 824

139. Menière's disease is characterized by:
    A. Vertigo   D. Nystagmus during an attack
    B. Hearing loss   E. All of the above
    C. Tinnitus   Ref. 2 - p. 623

140. Biochemical manifestations of Reye's disease includes all of
    the following, except:
    A. High elevation of serum transaminase
    B. Moderate increase in bilirubin
    C. Metabolic alkalosis
    D. Elevation of blood urea nitrogen
    E. Aminoaciduria   Ref. 11 - p. 888

141. Measures to prevent the propagation of Aedes aegypti are used
    to control:
    A. Malaria   D. Yellow fever
    B. Sleeping sickness   E. Rocky Mountain spotted
    C. Smallpox   fever
                                       Ref. 2 - p. 238

142. Which statement about esophageal cancer is false?
    A. Is usually of squamous cell type
    B. Most common in the distal portion
    C. Resection gives excellent results if followed by chemother-
       apy
    D. Primarily a disease of elderly males
    E. Characterized by dysphagia and painless weight loss
                                       Ref. 6 - p. 1036

143. Which of the following is not characteristic of hemolytic icterus?
    A. Pain and itching
    B. Increased fragility of erythrocytes
    C. Spherocytes in blood smear
    D. Hypercholic stools
    E. No increase in urinary pigment excretion
    Ref. 6 - p. 1001

144. Rectal prolapse in children less than 5 years old is best treated by:
    A. Thiersch wire
    B. Abdominal rectopexy (Ripstein procedure)
    C. No surgery; conservative followup
    D. Diverting colostomy
    E. High residue diet   Ref. 4 - p. 993

145. Epistaxis is most frequently caused by:
    A. Picking the nose   D. Sinusitis
    B. Adenoidal hypertrophy   E. Influenza
    C. Polyps   Ref. 11 - p. 937

146. Which one of the following statements regarding heat exhaustion is generally true?
    A. Water intoxication is usually present
    B. The illness is always fatal
    C. Anhidrosis is usually present
    D. Hypertension is a constant feature
    E. Marked elevation of body temperature usually occurs
    Ref. 2 - p. 65

147. The liver differs from most other organs in its:
    A. Lack of smooth muscle
    B. Being controlled by hormones
    C. Rich arterial supply
    D. Ability to regenerate
    E. Poor lymphatic drainage   Ref. 6 - p. 275

148. In over half the cases, acute bacterial infection of the middle ear is due to:
    A. Hemophilus influenzae   D. Staphylococci
    B. Streptococci   E. None of the above
    C. Diplococcus pneumoniae   Ref. 11 - p. 953

149. Bilirubin in plasma is tightly bound to:
    A. Albumin   D. Ceruloplasmin
    B. Gamma globulin   E. Haptoglobin
    C. Fibrinogen   Ref. 2 - p. 1324

150. Mature gametes have:
    A. 22 autosomes and 2 sex chromosomes
    B. Haploid number of chromosomes
    C. Diploid number of chromosomes
    D. All of the above
    E. None of the above   Ref. 7 - p. 108

151. In post-abortal infections exhibiting general sepsis, shock and renal failure, the most likely organism is:
    A. E. coli   D. Pseudomonas
    B. Clostridium welchii   E. Staphylococcus
    C. Proteus   Ref. 8 - p. 646

152. The serum antibody primarily responsible for fighting gram-positive pyogenic bacteria is:
    A. IgG   D. IgD
    B. IgA   E. IgE
    C. IgM   Ref. 1 - p. 346

153. There is an increased incidence of tubal pregnancy after:
    A. Chemotherapy for pelvic tuberculosis
    B. Chronic salpingitis
    C. Congenital tubal abnormalities
    D. A and B only
    E. All of the above   Ref. 8 - p. 566

154. Not characteristic of endometriosis is:
    A. Sterility
    B. Dyspareunia
    C. Progressive primary dysmenorrhea
    D. Nodular thickening of uterosacral ligaments
    E. Pain on defecation   Ref. 8 - p. 559

155. Bandl's pathological retraction ring:
    A. Characterized by marked thickening of lower uterine segment
    B. Is common with twins
    C. Is the same as the constriction ring
    D. Implies impending uterine rupture
    E. None of the above   Ref. 7 - p. 850

156. The incidence of salmonella infections is increased most often in patients with:
    A. Thalassemia major   D. Sickle cell disease
    B. Hereditary spherocytosis   E. Erythrocyte pyruvate kinase
    C. Hemoglobin C disease   deficiency
                                  Ref. 1 - p. 809

157. Measures useful in the treatment of hyperkalemia may include:
    A. Intravenous glucose and insulin
    B. Intravenous sodium bicarbonate
    C. Intravenous calcium chloride
    D. Oral or rectal Kayexelate
    E. All of the above   Ref. 2 - p. 1589

158. Hypertrophic osteoarthropathy:
    A. May serve as an indicator of pulmonary neoplasms
    B. On radiological examination may reveal periosteal new bone
       formation
    C. May be painful
    D. Is often associated with clubbing of the fingers
    E. All of the above are true   Ref. 2 - p. 1843

159. Evidence of monoclonal protein production in multiple myeloma
    may be detected:
    A. In the serum in 80% of cases
    B. In the serum and urine in 20% of cases
    C. In the urine alone in 20% of cases
    D. None of the above
    E. All of the above   Ref. 1 - p. 355

160. The Stein-Leventhal syndrome may be associated with:
    A. Ovarian malignancy   D. Endometrial carcinoma
    B. Hypopituitarism   E. Cervical dysplasia
    C. Adrenal cortical hyperplasia   Ref. 8 - p. 347

161. The most common form of croup is:
    A. Acute spasmodic laryngitis   D. Acute laryngotracheobron-
    B. Acute infectious laryngitis   chitis
    C. Acute epiglottitis   E. Hypocalcemic tetany
                                        Ref. 11 - p. 962

162. Causes of anal fissures include all of the following except:
    A. Idiopathic   D. Syphilis
    B. Crohn's disease   E. Gonorrhea
    C. Carcinoma of anal canal   Ref. 4 - p. 1000

163. In idiopathic hypopituitarism all of the following laboratory re-
    sults are usually obtained, except:
    A. High serum Na   D. Low 24-hour RAI uptake
    B. Low serum Na   E. Low blood glucose
    C. Low PBI   Ref. 2 - p. 1692

164. Each of the following drugs may precipitate hemolysis in a
    patient with glucose 6-phosphate dehydrogenase deficiency,
    except:
    A. Prednisone   D. Phenacetin
    B. Nitrofurantoin   E. Vitamin K substitutes
    C. Acetyisalicylic acid   Ref. 1 - p. 1599

165. Hypokalemia may be commonly produced by each one of the following diuretic agents, except:
    A. Mercuhydrin   D. Triamterene
    B. Hydrochlorothiazide E. Furosemide
    C. Ethacrynic acid   Ref. 1 - p. 1125

166. Thyroid hyperplasia is due to all, except:
    A. Iodine-deficient diet
    B. Increased secretion of TSH
    C. Stimulation from the adrenal gland
    D. Thyroid-blocking drugs or dietary substances
    E. None of the above
                                Ref. 6 - p. 1433

167. Benign monoclonal gammopathy is characterized by:
    A. Homogeneous serum spike and 90% plasma cells in the marrow
    B. Homogeneous serum spike, anemia and absence of bone lesions
    C. Homogeneous serum spike and slight increase in plasma cells
    D. Homogeneous serum spike and excellent response to therapy
    E. None of the above   Ref. 1 - p. 356

168. Chronic prostatitis may be based on any of the following, except:
    A. Instrumentation   D. Retrograde infection from
    B. Congestion and stasis   urethra
    C. Distant foci of infection E. Syphilis or tuberculosis
                                Ref. 6 - p. 1560

169. Each of the following statements regarding E. coli infections is true, except:
    A. They commonly cause urinary tract infections
    B. Subcutaneous abscesses may be characterized by gas formation
    C. They are a common cause of pharyngitis in newborn children
    D. Some strains are sensitive to tetracycline
    E. Some strains are sensitive to kanamycin
                                Ref. 1 - p. 792

170. All of the following are true of placenta previa, except:
    A. Higher incidence in women with low segment C-section
    B. Premature labor is common
    C. Malposition and malpresentation are common
    D. First trimester bleeding is not uncommon
    E. Postpartum hemorrhage is infrequent
                                Ref. 7 - pp. 609-618

171. Each of the following statements regarding salicylate poisoning
is true, except:
A. It is more common in children
B. Respiratory alkalosis may occur
C. Metabolic alkalosis may occur
D. Metabolic acidosis may occur
E. Sodium bicarbonate may be useful in therapy
Ref. 2 - p. 57

172. All of the following are characteristic of staphylococcal pneu-
monia, except:
A. Incidence highest during winter months
B. Usually preceded by a viral upper respiratory infection
C. Found most commonly in infants
D. Rapid progression of symptoms is common
E. Radiographic evidence of bronchopneumonia usually does
not appear until late in the illness
Ref. 11 - pp. 972-973

173. Each of the following statements regarding paroxysmal noctur-
nal hemoglobinuria is true, except:
A. It appears to be an acquired disorder
B. It is seen commonly following a syphilitic infection
C. The acidified serum test (Ham's test) is often positive
D. Pancytopenia is often a feature of the illness
E. Symptoms often develop during sleep
Ref. 1 - p. 1609

174. The left lobe of the liver is defined by:
A. The falciform ligament
B. The porta hepatis
C. A line between the gallbladder bed and the inferior vena cava
D. A line between the portal vein and the falciform ligament
E. A line between the portal vein and the inferior vena cava
Ref. 4 - p. 1007

175. Examples of transudates in the pleural cavity usually include
each of the following, except:
A. Congestive heart failure   D. Nephritis
B. Empyema   E. Meigs' syndrome
C. Cirrhosis of the liver   Ref. 1 - p. 1327

176. Mediastinal neoplasms must be differentiated from the follow-
ing, except:
A. Esophageal dilatation
B. Aneurysm
C. Lesions of sternum or vertebrae
D. Lymphoma
E. Diaphragmatic hernia   Ref. 6 - p. 663

177. Cryoglobulinemia may be found in association with:
    A. Multiple myeloma
    B. Systemic lupus erythematosus
    C. In apparently healthy individuals
    D. All of the above
    E. None of the above   Ref. 1 - p. 358

178. All are true of gangrene of the uterus, except:
    A. A rare and grave form of puerperal infection
    B. Endometrium undergoes necrosis
    C. Myometrium undergoes necrosis
    D. Characterized by expulsion of large pieces of necrotic material
    E. Usually occurs the second postpartum day
                                  Ref. 7 - p. 982

179. Increased plasma concentrations of each of the following is usually found in severe renal failure, except:
    A. Phosphorus   D. Uric acid
    B. Calcium   E. Sulfate
    C. Creatinine   Ref. 2 - p. 1099

180. All of the following cardiac catheterization pressures are expected in patent ductus arteriosus, except:
    A. Venae cavae-normal
    B. Right atrium-markedly elevated
    C. Right ventricle-normal to increased
    D. Pulmonary artery-normal to increased
    E. Pulmonary capillary-normal to increased
                                  Ref. 11 - p. 1012

181. Each of the following enzyme deficiencies is associated with hemolytic anemia, except:
    A. Glucose 6-phosphate dehydrogenase
    B. Pyruvate kinase
    C. Glucose 6-phosphatase
    D. Triosephosphate isomerase
    E. Hexokinase   Ref. 1 - p. 1602

182. Symptoms of acute prostatitis include all, except:
    A. Urethral discharge
    B. Burning on urination
    C. Increased frequency of urination
    D. Pain in the pelvis or perineum
    E. Incontinence   Ref. 6 - p. 1560

183. Each of the following statements regarding the Wolff-Parkinson-White syndrome is true, except:
    A. The configuration of P-waves is normal
    B. The P-R interval is usually more than 0. 22 sec
    C. The QRS interval is usually increased

D. A slur in the initial phase of the QRS complex is often present (delta wave)
E. Propranolol may be effective during an attack of tachycardia
Ref. 1 - p. 1142

184. The hepatic artery supplies approximately ____% of blood flow to the liver.
A. 10%   D. 75%
B. 25%   E. 90%
C. 50%   Ref. 6 - p. 1178

185. Each of the following is characteristic of a villous adenoma of the rectum, except:
A. Diarrhea   D. Large, sessile growth
B. Rectal bleeding   E. Frequent diagnosis by sig-
C. Hyperkalemia   moidoscopy
                         Ref. 2 - pp. 1302, 1587

186. All of the following are characteristics of the female pelvis, except:
A. Symphysis pubis is wide and shallow
B. Suprapubic angle acute
C. True pelvis shallow and wide
D. Bones are light and graceful in structure
E. Sacrosciatic notch is wide   Ref. 7 - pp. 313-316

187. In male patients with severe liver disease, each of the following is commonly observed, except:
A. Reduced libido   D. Decrease in secondary sex
B. Impotence   characteristics
C. Gynecomastia   E. Increase in axillary hair
                           Ref. 2 - p. 1328

188. In simple valvular pulmonic stenosis:
A. There is an increase in systolic pressure
B. There is hypertrophy of the right ventricle
C. Pulmonary artery pressure is low or normal
D. Arterial oxygen saturation is normal
E. All of the above   Ref. 11 - p. 1054

Each group of questions below consists of lettered headings followed by a list of numbered words or phrases. For each numbered word or phrase select the one heading which is most closely related to it:

Match the following:

A. The angle that the plane of the superior pelvic strait forms with the horizon
B. 11 cm
C. 10.5 cm
D. 12.5 cm
E. An imaginary line which passes through the center of any pelvic plane

189. ___ Conjugata vera
190. ___ Obstetrical conjugate
191. ___ Diagonal conjugate
192. ___ Pelvic inclination
193. ___ Pelvic axis   Ref. 7 - pp. 290-296

Regarding differential diagnosis of acute pancreatitis:

A. Perforated peptic ulcer
B. Acute peptic ulcer
C. Small bowel obstruction
D. Colon obstruction
E. Acute pancreatitis

194. ___ Tender, palpable RUQ mass
195. ___ Crampy, colicky pain and distinctive X-ray film
196. ___ Free air under diaphragm
197. ___ Elevated serum amylase
198. ___ Painless distention and distinctive X-ray film
                    Ref. 6 - pp. 967-972

A. Decrease in polymorphonuclear leukocytes
B. Decrease in eosinophils
C. Increase in monocytes
D. Increase in basophils
E. Increase in eosinophils

199. ___ Noted in pemphigus, allergic states and Hodgkin's disease
200. ___ Noted in myeloproliferative diseases
201. ___ Commonly produced by thiouracil
202. ___ Often associated with tuberculosis
203. ___ Result of corticosteroid therapy
                    Ref. 1 - pp. 318, 320, 321

A. Ichthyosis vulgaris
B. Epidermolytic hyperkeratosis
C. Psoriasis
D. Seborrheic dermatitis
E. Leiner's disease

204. ___ Blisters, background erythema, flexural involvement, lesions frequently present at birth, may abate spontaneously after puberty
205. ___ Dryness and scaling on extensor surfaces, onset after age 3 months, hyperkeratosis, treatment is topical and symptomatic
206. ___ Relatively common, onset common before age 10 years, red plaques surrounded by a silvery-white scale, etiology unknown
207. ___ Erythema with yellowish greasy-appearing scales usually localized to scalp, eyebrows, nasolabial folds and presternal skin
208. ___ Generalized erythema, subsequent shedding of skin, confined to infancy, a generalized exfoliative dermatitis
Ref. 10 - pp. 1755-1759

A. Bacterial meningitis
B. Syphilis
C. Carcinomatous meningitis
D. Subdural empyema
E. Bacterial endocarditis

209. ___ Reduced sugar and mononuclear pleocytosis
210. ___ High pressure, normal sugar, protein 100-500
211. ___ Glucose less than 40, with protein 100-500
212. ___ Normal pressure, normal sugar, mixed increase in polys lymphs
213. ___ High gamma globulin and lymphocyte pleocytosis
Ref. 2 - pp. 670-671

Match mediastinal mass with area in which found:

A. Superior mediastinum
B. Anterior mediastinum
C. Posterior mediastinum
D. Not specific

214. ___ Dermoids and teratomas
215. ___ Bronchogenic cyst
216. ___ Intrathoracic goiter
217. ___ Metastatic cancer
218. ___ Thymic mass   Ref. 6 - p. 664

Match the following:

A. Secretin
B. Pancreozymin
C. Both
D. Neither

219. ___ Also known as cholecystokinin
220. ___ Increases volume of pancreatic secretion
221. ___ Increases enzyme content of pancreatic secretion
222. ___ Increase bicarbonate content of pancreatic secretion
223. ___ Action potentiated by vagal stimulation

Ref. 4 - pp. 1099-1100

A. Gonococcal conjunctivitis
B. Inclusion blennorrhea
C. Allergic conjunctivitis, simple
D. Membranous conjunctivitis
E. Epidemic keratoconjunctivitis

224. ___ Caused by a filterable virus transmitted from genital tract of mother during delivery, acute onset, mucopurulent exudate, photophobia, treat with sulfonamides
225. ___ Hyperemia, edema, profuse lacrimation, severe itching
226. ___ Infection usually bilateral, generally appears on 2nd or 3rd day of life
227. ___ Acute, contagious disease of conjunctiva, caused by adenovirus type 8, rapid onset of acute follicular conjunctivitis
228. ___ May be associated with Stevens-Johnson syndrome, may cause significant change to conjunctiva and cornea

Ref. 10 - pp. 1819-1821

A. Vitamin B_{12}
B. Folic acid
C. Vitamin D
D. Iron
E. Calcium

229. ___ Present in the diet in a conjugated form
230. ___ Intestinal absorption is facilitated by parathyroid hormone
231. ___ Absorption dependent upon presence of "intrinsic factor"
232. ___ Absorption occurs in the duodenum and is diminished in the presence of achlorhydria
233. ___ Fat soluble

Ref. 2 - p. 1219

Match the following:

A. Parotid gland
B. Submaxillary gland
C. Both
D. Neither

234. ___ Most tumors of this gland are benign
235. ___ Most tumors of this gland are malignant
236. ___ Most salivary gland tumors occur here
237. ___ Facial nerve passes through this gland
238. ___ Site of Warthin's tumor   Ref. 4 - p. 1268

Match urinary pH with associated stone type:

A. Acid urine
B. Alkaline urine
C. Not pH dependant

239. ___ Calcium oxalate
240. ___ Triple phosphate
241. ___ Uric acid
242. ___ Cystine
243. ___ Foreign body   Ref. 4 - p. 1505

A. Visceral larva migrans
B. Enterobiasis
C. Hookworm disease
D. Trichinosis
E. Bancroft's filariasis

244. ___ Perianal pruritis, treated with piperazine
245. ___ Parasite found in small intestine of man, larva penetrates skin, diagnosis made by observing eggs in feces
246. ___ Early symptoms include diarrhea, fever, eosinophilia and periorbital edema
247. ___ Toxocara canis, transmitted by ingestion of eggs from soil
248. ___ Located in lymphatics and lymph nodes, treated with Diethyl-carbamazine   Ref. 10 - p. 798

A. Gumma
B. Optic atrophy
C. Tabes dorsalis
D. Meningovascular syphilis
E. Meningitis

249. ___ Gastric or visceral crises leading to unnecessary surgery
250. ___ Headache, wide variety of neurologic deficits, and excellent posterior column function
251. ___ Behaves as a slowly growing CNS mass
252. ___ Occurs during the early weeks of syphilitic infection
253. ___ Blacks are more prone to develop this form of neurosyphilis than whites   Ref. 2 - pp. 680-683

A. Placenta previa
B. Abruptio placenta
C. Both
D. Neither

254. ___ Common source of third trimester hemorrhage
255. ___ Bleeding may be occult
256. ___ Associated with DIC
257. ___ Associated with abnormal fetal presentations
258. ___ Associated with hypertensive disorders of pregnancy
Ref. 7 - pp. 609-635

A. Pulmonary stenosis
B. Tetralogy of Fallot
C. Both
D. Neither

259. ___ Loud systolic murmur heard in neck
260. ___ Dyspnea
261. ___ Cardiac failure very rare
262. ___ Cerebrovascular accident
263. ___ Heart normal in size, rate and rhythm
Ref. 6 - p. 723

A. Osteomalacia
B. Paget's disease of bone
C. Both
D. Neither

264. ___ Bone pain
265. ___ Tetany
266. ___ Low serum alkaline phosphatase
267. ___ Cardiac failure
268. ___ Pseudofractures   Ref. 1 - pp. 1974, 1969

A. Goodpasture's syndrome
B. Idiopathic pulmonary hemosiderosis
C. Both
D. Neither

269. ___ Hemoptysis
270. ___ Nephritis
271. ___ Nodular pulmonary infiltrates by X-ray
272. ___ Prognosis excellent
273. ___ Adrenal steroids are often curative
Ref. 2 - p. 853

A. Hepatogenous jaundice
B. Obstructive jaundice
C. Both
D. Neither

274. ___ Usually a surgical case
275. ___ Thymol turbidity test positive
276. ___ Pain in 80% of cases
277. ___ Primarily in young adults
278. ___ More intense jaundice   Ref. 6 - p. 1001

     A. Hydronephrosis
     B. Wilms' tumor
     C. Both
     D. Neither

279. ___ Painless mass
280. ___ Intravenous pyelogram is diagnostic
281. ___ Usually based at ureteropelvic junction
282. ___ Excellent long-term results from operation
283. ___ More often bilateral   Ref. 6 - p. 1567

     A. Pituitary apoplexy
     B. Craniopharyngioma
     C. Chromophobe adenoma
     D. Eosinophilic adenoma
     E. Empty sella syndrome

284. ___ Most common pituitary tumor
285. ___ Benign condition caused by increased intracranial pressure
286. ___ May occur spontaneously or after radiation
287. ___ The position of this tumor is usually suprasellar
288. ___ Prognathism is one of the characteristic results
                       Ref. 1 - pp. 447-449

Match the following:

     A. Glioblastoma multiforme
     B. Medulloblastoma
     C. Posterior fossa
     D. Anterior fossa

289. ___ Most common brain tumor in adults
290. ___ Most common brain tumor in children
291. ___ Most malignant type of brain tumor
292. ___ Most common site of brain tumor in adults
293. ___ Most common site of brain tumor in children
                       Ref. 4 - p. 1279

     A. Extradural hematoma
     B. Subdural hematoma
     C. Both
     D. Neither

294. ___ Usually due to a tear in middle meningeal artery
295. ___ 85% in children 1 year of age or younger

296. ___ Most lethal complication of head injury, untreated mortality 100%
297. ___ Typical clinical syndrome apparent in first 12 to 24 hours
298. ___ Initial presenting sign is a focal seizure

Ref. 10 - pp. 970-971

A. Polymyositis
B. Duchenne muscular dystrophy
C. Both
D. Neither

299. ___ Equal sex distribution
300. ___ Rapid rate of progression
301. ___ Marked muscular atrophy
302. ___ Spontaneous remission is the rule
303. ___ No response to cortisone   Ref. 10 - p. 1033

A. Rocky Mountain spotted fever
B. Murine typhus
C. Both
D. Neither

304. ___ Rickettsia
305. ___ Centripetal rash
306. ___ Centrifugal rash
307. ___ Chloramphenicol
308. ___ Positive Weil-Felix reaction   Ref. 1 - pp. 913, 917

After each of the following case histories there is a series of multiple choice questions based on the history. Select the one most appropriate answer:

CASE(Questions 309-312): A 45-year-old male complains of abdominal pain, diarrhea and wheezing of several months duration. Questioning reveals that the patient experiences peculiar episodes of blurred vision and flushing of the face after a heavy meal. On physical examination, abnormal findings include facial telangiectasia, hepatomegaly, darkening of the skin and a heart murmur.

309. The skin of the patient is most likely to resemble that of individuals with:
A. Scurvy
B. Porphyria
C. Hemochromatosis
D. Pellagra
E. Addison's disease

310. The heart murmur is most likely to sound like:
A. Mitral stenosis
B. Atrial septal defect
C. Mitral insufficiency
D. Pulmonic stenosis
E. Tetralogy of Fallot

311. Which of the following would be most useful in arriving at a diagnosis?
   A. D-xylose absorption
   B. Urinary excretion of 5-hydroxyindolacetic acid
   C. Urinary excretion of VMA
   D. Urinary excretion of ALA
   E. Urinary excretion of 17-hydroxycorticosteroids

312. A false positive test for this disorder might result if a normal individual had previously eaten a diet high in:
   A. Nuts
   B. Bananas
   C. Monosodium glutamate
   D. Seafood
   E. Polyunsaturated fatty acids
   Ref. 2 - p. 1796, 1798

CASE (Questions 313-316): A 59-year-old woman has had an asymptomatic mass in the lower neck for 20 years. Four years ago the mass began to enlarge and recently there has been a choking sensation. There have been no eye changes, no pulse elevation and no weight loss.

313. The differential includes all, except:
   A. Fetal adenoma
   B. Cystic hygroma
   C. Nontoxic nodular goiter
   D. Thyroid cancer
   E. Thyroiditis

314. Treatment is indicated because of all, except:
   A. Mass may be malignant or become so
   B. Esophageal obstruction should be relieved
   C. Cosmetic reasons require it
   D. Threat of future thyroiditis
   E. Thyrotoxicosis may develop later

315. Preferred treatment in this case is:
   A. Subtotal thyroidectomy
   B. X-ray therapy
   C. Iodine and desiccated thyroid
   D. Antithyroid drugs
   E. Radioisotope

316. Complications of treatment may include any, except:
   A. Recurrent nerve injury
   B. Hypoparathyroidism
   C. Recurrent nodules in lateral lymph nodes
   D. Myxedema
   E. Tracheal collapse
   Ref. 6 - p. 1446

CASE (Questions 317-320): A 3-year-old boy has had a severe cough almost since birth and with great difficulty brings up extremely tenacious sputum of ropy character. There have been episodes of high fever, and labored respiration, with slight cyanosis.

317. The suspected diagnosis is:
   A. Sequestered lung
   B. Tuberculosis
   C. Mucoviscidosis
   D. Small tracheoesophageal fistula
   E. Bronchiectasis

318. The diagnosis is established by:
   A. Chest X-ray for detection of emphysema
   B. Test for sodium loss in sweat
   C. Secretin test of pancreatic function
   D. Sputum examination for organisms and cells
   E. Differential spirometry

319. Early treatment is essential to avoid all, except:
   A. Chronic bronchitis
   B. Bronchiectasis
   C. Bronchial hemorrhage
   D. Emphysema
   E. Pulmonary fibrosis

320. Which statement is false in regard to regimen of therapy?
   A. Mucolytic agents should be inhaled or instilled
   B. Antibiotics are necessary to control infection in atelectatic areas
   C. Postural drainage is useful after mucolytic agents are used
   D. Surgical excision of all bronchiectatic areas is important
   E. Pancreatic extract helps control the basic pancreatic insufficiency   Ref. 6 - p. 634

CASE (Questions 321-324): Two hours previously, an 18-year-old primigravida was delivered by low forceps and midline episiotomy. A large bluish mass now involves the perineal body.

321. What is the most likely diagnosis?
   A. Ruptured vulvar varix
   B. Hematoma formation
   C. Thrombosed hemorrhoid
   D. Bruised episiotomy site
   E. None of the above

322. The best treatment for the situation above is:
   A. Observation
   B. Transfusion
   C. Incision and evacuation
   D. Vaginal tamponade
   E. Ice to perineum

323. In addition the above therapy should also include:
   A. Fibrinogen
   B. Antibiotics
   C. Calcium gluconate
   D. Anticoagulants
   E. Plasma

324. The first symptom most often noted is:
    A. Excruciating pain by the patient
    B. Shock
    C. Necrosis of skin overlying the lesion
    D. Infection
    E. Anemia   Ref. 7 - pp. 999-1000

CASE (Questions 325-328): A 10-month-old infant has been in good
health but suddenly cries out with "abdominal colic." Several episodes
occur within a three-hour period, some accompanied by vomiting.
The youngster appears quite ill. A physician attends the child and
during his examination, the infant passes some blood and mucous
per rectum. On examination there are obvious signs of ileus, dis-
tension-vomiting-tachycardia. The abdomen appears to be non-tender.

325. The most likely diagnosis is:
    A. Volvulus   D. Diverticulitis
    B. Acute appendicitis   E. Ruptured spleen
    C. Intussusception

326. In most cases the initial symptom is:
    A. Abdominal pain   D. Dehydration
    B. Bloody stools   E. Anorexia
    C. Lethargy

327. The "best" description of the stool in this disorder is:
    A. Rice water   D. Seedy
    B. Currant jelly   E. Tarry
    C. Black water

328. An uncommon physical finding, associated with this disorder:
    A. Apathetic or prostrated child D. Palpable mass
    B. Fever of 101° F   E. Petechiae
    C. Elevated pulse   Ref. 10 - pp. 1654-1658

CASE (Questions 329-332): A 35-year-old female was seen because
of anorexia, weakness and weight loss of 20 pounds in the past month.
The patient has been known to have rheumatic heart disease for
several years. In the past two weeks she had noticed that she was
short of breath on moderate exertion and that her legs were swollen.
She had a temperature of 101° F. Her pulse was 110/min and irregular. The cardiac examination revealed a diastolic murmur at the
apex. There were several petechial lesions around the right clavicle,
and the splenic tip was palpable. She had a tooth extraction one month
ago.

329. The most probable diagnosis is:
    A. Miliary tuberculosis   D. Subacute bacterial endo-
    B. German measles   carditis
    C. Recurrent rheumatic fever E. Sickle cell anemia

330. Which one of the following procedures is most helpful in the diagnosis and management of her illness?
    A. Blood cultures and sensitivity
    B. Sputum culture for AFB
    C. Hemoglobin electrophoresis
    D. Lymph node biopsy
    E. Culture and sensitivity of a pharyngeal swab

331. Which one of the following findings is not usually a manifestation of her illness?
    A. Roth spots
    B. Bitot spots
    C. Janeway spots
    D. Osler's nodes
    E. Splinter hemorrhages

332. The complications of her illness may include:
    A. Cerebral embolus
    B. Splenic infarct
    C. "Flea-bitten kidney"
    D. Mycotic aneurysms
    E. All of the above
    Ref. 2 - p. 310

CASE (Questions 333-336): A 58-year-old carpenter had noted a nodular thickening in his right palm in the region of the distal palmar crease over the fourth metacarpophalangeal joint. Then a firm cord, thought to be the tendon, appeared at the base of the ring finger which gradually assumed a flexed position.

333. Your diagnosis is:
    A. Sclerosing tenosynovitis
    B. Volkmann's contracture
    C. Dupuytren's contracture
    D. Tuberculous tendonitis
    E. Traumatic tenosynovitis

334. The seat of pathologic change here is in:
    A. Palmar aponeurosis
    B. Tendon sheath
    C. Tendon
    D. Subcutaneous fat
    E. Deep layers of palmar skin

335. Treatment is best accomplished by:
    A. Tendon lengthening
    B. Z-plasty to the skin
    C. X-ray to disperse fibrous tissue
    D. Fasciotomy
    E. Cortisone to abolish fibrosis

336. Which statement regarding fasciotomy is false?
    A. Limited fasciotomy usually leads to recurrence
    B. Radical fasciotomy carries too much risk to vessels and nerves
    C. Removal of all palmar fascia under tourniquet is best
    D. Zigzag incision and Z-plasty closure prevents skin contracture
    E. Hand is dressed with fingers partially flexed to avoid gangrene-producing tension of the suture line
    Ref. 6 - p. 1715

CASE (Questions 337-340): An 18-year-old nulliparous female is admitted to the hospital with a semi-solid 5 cm pelvic mass. There have been no menstrual abnormalities or disturbances in bowel or bladder function. Her last menstrual period began 10 days ago. The only symptoms have been vague lower abdominal pain. On pelvic exam the mass is found to be mobile and anterior to the uterus. The rest of the pelvic examination as well as her general physical exam is normal.

337. The most likely diagnosis is:
   A. Corpus luteum cyst
   B. Benign teratoma (dermoid)
   C. Granulosa cell tumor
   D. Arrhenoblastoma
   E. Endometrioma of ovary
      Ref. 8 - pp. 460-464

338. The incidence of this tumor in the opposite ovary is:
   A. 11%
   B. 50%
   C. 25%
   D. 0%
   E. 75%
      Ref. 8 - pp. 460-464

339. X-ray picture of the abdomen is likely to show:
   A. Nothing
   B. Teeth
   C. Psammoma bodies
   D. Reinke crystals
   E. Phleboliths
      Ref. 8 - pp. 460-464

340. The incidence of a malignancy occurring in this type of tumor is:
   A. 0
   B. 1%
   C. 5%
   D. 10%
   E. 15%
      Ref. 8 - pp. 460-464

CASE (Questions 341-344): A 25-year-old female complains of frequent headaches in the temporal regions for about 5 years. All her four sisters and her mother used to have similar complaints. Just prior to an attack, she complains of blind spots and intense nausea. Her entire physical examination is negative.

341. The most probable cause of her headaches is:
   A. Cluster headaches
   B. Brain tumor
   C. Subarachnoid hemorrhage
   D. Myopia
   E. Migraine

342. During an acute attack increased excretion of _____ may be found in the urine:
   A. Epinephrine
   B. Calcium
   C. Serotonin metabolites
   D. Phosphorus
   E. Urobilinogen

343. The attacks frequently respond to:
   A. Estrogen
   B. Cortisone
   C. Methysergide
   D. Craniotomy
   E. Corrective eye glasses

344. A complication of the above therapy may include:
    A. Hirsutism   D. Retroperitoneal fibrosis
    B. Focal epilepsy   E. Sterility
    C. Iridocyclitis   Ref. 2 - pp. 616,1078

CASE (Questions 345-348): A 10-year-old boy has been known to have a cardiac murmur since birth. He was never cyanotic. Recently he has developed exertional dyspnea. On examination there was a loud systolic murmur at the second left intercostal area. The second heart sound was widely split and not fixed. The pulmonic component of the second sound was diminished in intensity. EKG revealed right ventricular hypertrophy.

345. The most probable diagnosis is:
    A. Interatrial septal defect   D. Pulmonic stenosis
    B. Interventricular septal defect E. Patent ductus arteriosus
    C. Aortic stenosis

346. The jugular venous pulse tracing is likely to show:
    A. Prominent A wave   D. Absence of V wave
    B. Prominent C wave   E. None of the above
    C. Absence of A wave

347. X-ray of the chest is likely to show:
    A. Increased prominence of pulmonary vascular markings
    B. Oligemic pulmonary vasculature
    C. Left ventricular hypertrophy
    D. Straightening of the left border of the heart
    E. Uncoiling of the aorta

348. Cardiac catheterization will probably reveal increased:
    A. Left atrial pressure   D. Pulmonary artery pressure
    B. Left ventricular pressure   E. Pulmonary artery wedge
    C. Right ventricular pressure   pressure
                                       Ref. 2 - p. 942

CASE (Questions 349-352): A 65-year-old man has survived a 55% body surface full-thickness burn for three weeks. The eschar is firm and dry.

349. It is now the time to:
    A. Stop the antibiotics
    B. Excise the eschar and do skin grafting
    C. Begin active exercises to small joints
    D. Check kidney function
    E. Do bacterial skin counts

350. Which type of coverage is preferred here after excising the eschar?
    A. Split thickness autografts
    B. Preserved calk dermis

    C. Split thickness homografts
    D. Pinch or postage stamp grafts
    E. Full-thickness flaps or pedicles

351. Which of the following is an advantage of homografting as a
     biological dressing?
    A. Serves to prevent loss of heat and water
    B. Quickly causes disappearance of surface bacteria
    C. Gives respite from pain and obviates dressing changes
    D. The donor problem is solved by cadaver skin
    E. All of the above

352. Which of the following regarding homografting in this case is
     false?
    A. The victim would not have sufficient skin for autografting
    B. No anesthesia is required for homografting
    C. Homografts grow rapidly to make a permanent covering
    D. The procedure reduces mortality from shock and infection
    E. Homografting allows 3 to 12 weeks to arrange for permanent
       coverage   Ref. 6 - p. 266-267

CASE (Questions 353-356): A 30-year-old man is brought into the
hospital in shock after an automobile accident. The only evident injury is a contusion on the left side of the head. The patient was awake
and responsive in the ambulance but lapsed into coma in the emergency room.

353. This patient's shock is most likely due to:
    A. Cerebral concussion   D. Deep intracerebral bleed
    B. Subdural hematoma   E. Extracranial injury
    C. Epidural hematoma   Ref. 4 - p. 1290

354. The priorities of treatment,in order, are:
    A. Start intravenous, skull x-rays, lumbar puncture, no sur-
       gery
    B. Secure airway, start intravenous, combat shock, cerebral
       angiogram, to O.R. for burr holes
    C. Secure airway, start intravenous, lumbar puncture, take
       to O.R. for burr holes
    D. Secure airway, start intravenous, combat shock, lumbar
       puncture, echoencephalogram, EEG
    E. Secure airway, start intravenous, combat shock, to O.R.
       for burr holes   Ref. 4 - p. 1290

355. The history of a "lucid interval" is most often associated with:
    A. Acute subdural bleed   D. Deep intracerebral bleed
    B. Berry aneurysm   E. Chronic subdural hematoma
    C. Acute epidural bleed   Ref. 4 - p. 1292

356. If this patient were found to have an epidural bleed, which artery is most likely involved?
   A. Superficial temporal
   B. Anterior cerebral
   C. Middle cerebral
   D. Middle meningeal
   E. Basilar
   Ref. 4 - p. 1292

For each of the questions or incomplete statements below, one or more of the answers or completions given is correct. Answer according to the following key:

   A. If only 1, 2 and 3 are correct
   B. If only 1 and 3 are correct
   C. If only 2 and 4 are correct
   D. If only 4 is correct
   E. If all are correct

357. Immediate treatment of the common bile duct injured at operation may be by which of the following?
   1. Direct suture of the duct
   2. Choledochoduodenostomy
   3. T-tube insertion
   4. Penrose drain insertion
   Ref. 6 - p. 1232

358. Which of the following factors predispose to duodenojejunal angle obstruction?
   1. Afferent loop syndrome
   2. Congenital malrotation
   3. Duodenal diverticula
   4. Thoracolumbar scoliosis
   Ref. 6 - p. 1525

359. Renovascular hypertension is associated with:
   1. Men more often affected than women
   2. Late filling of affected side on IVP
   3. Decreased creatinine concentration on affected side
   4. Hyperconcentration of IVP dye on affected side
   Ref. 4 - p. 1521

360. Some degree of fecal incontinence tends to remain after successful repair of long-standing rectal prolapse in the adult because:
   1. Pelvic floor structures are severely relaxed
   2. Patient is accustomed to being soiled
   3. Constipation continues to be a problem
   4. The anal sphincter is chronically stretched
   Ref. 6 - p. 1156

ANSWER KEY

1. B	51. D	101. E	151. B	201. A
2. D	52. A	102. D	152. A	202. C
3. C	53. D	103. B	153. E	203. B
4. B	54. D	104. C	154. C	204. B
5. A	55. B	105. B	155. D	205. A
6. B	56. C	106. D	156. D	206. C
7. D	57. C	107. E	157. E	207. D
8. E	58. D	108. D	158. E	208. E
9. D	59. A	109. E	159. E	209. C
10. B	60. A	110. A	160. D	210. D
11. C	61. C	111. B	161. D	211. A
12. C	62. C	112. E	162. E	212. E
13. D	63. D	113. B	163. A	213. B
14. E	64. C	114. B	164. A	214. B
15. B	65. C	115. E	165. D	215. C
16. E	66. D	116. C	166. C	216. A
17. D	67. B	117. C	167. C	217. D
18. B	68. E	118. A	168. E	218. B
19. A	69. E	119. E	169. C	219. B
20. C	70. D	120. A	170. E	220. A
21. E	71. E	121. D	171. C	221. B
22. B	72. D	122. D	172. E	222. A
23. E	73. E	123. D	173. B	223. C
24. A	74. E	124. C	174. C	224. B
25. A	75. C	125. B	175. B	225. C
26. D	76. D	126. B	176. D	226. A
27. C	77. E	127. D	177. D	227. E
28. A	78. D	128. B	178. E	228. D
29. C	79. B	129. C	179. B	229. B
30. E	80. D	130. A	180. B	230. E
31. B	81. A	131. A	181. C	231. A
32. C	82. D	132. D	182. E	232. D
33. A	83. E	133. B	183. B	233. C
34. E	84. B	134. B	184. B	234. A
35. C	85. D	135. A	185. C	235. B
36. A	86. C	136. E	186. B	236. A
37. E	87. E	137. B	187. E	237. A
38. C	88. A	138. D	188. E	238. A
39. A	89. C	139. E	189. B	239. C
40. A	90. A	140. C	190. C	240. B
41. D	91. D	141. D	191. D	241. A
42. C	92. D	142. C	192. A	242. A
43. B	93. D	143. A	193. E	243. C
44. C	94. C	144. C	194. B	244. B
45. C	95. A	145. A	195. C	245. C
46. E	96. D	146. C	196. A	246. D
47. C	97. D	147. D	197. E	247. A
48. A	98. C	148. C	198. D	248. E
49. C	99. C	149. A	199. E	249. C
50. B	100. D	150. B	200. D	250. D

ANSWER KEY

251. A	301. B	351. E
252. E	302. D	352. C
253. B	303. B	353. E
254. C	304. C	354. B
255. B	305. B	355. C
256. B	306. A	356. D
257. A	307. C	357. B
258. B	308. C	358. C
259. A	309. D	359. C
260. C	310. D	360. D
261. B	311. B	
262. B	312. B	
263. B	313. B	
264. C	314. D	
265. A	315. A	
266. D	316. C	
267. B	317. C	
268. A	318. B	
269. C	319. C	
270. A	320. D	
271. C	321. B	
272. D	322. C	
273. D	323. B	
274. B	324. A	
275. A	325. C	
276. B	326. A	
277. A	327. B	
278. A	328. E	
279. B	329. D	
280. C	330. A	
281. A	331. B	
282. D	332. E	
283. A	333. C	
284. C	334. A	
285. E	335. D	
286. A	336. B	
287. B	337. B	
288. D	338. C	
289. A	339. B	
290. B	340. B	
291. A	341. E	
292. D	342. C	
293. C	343. C	
294. A	344. D	
295. B	345. D	
296. A	346. A	
297. A	347. B	
298. D	348. C	
299. D	349. B	
300. A	350. C	

THIRD EXAMINATION

For each of the following multiple choice questions, select the one most appropriate answer:

1. Manifestations of general paresis often include:
   A. Megalomania
   B. Euphoria
   C. Dementia
   D. CSF examination which is always abnormal
   E. All of the above
   Ref. 2 - p. 681

2. Drug-induced parkinsonism may be caused by:
   A. Cortisone
   B. Nitrofurantoin
   C. Phenothiazines
   D. Levophed
   E. Scopolamine
   Ref. 2 - p. 637

3. Spinbarkeit is a term which means:
   A. Crystallization of cervical mucus
   B. Threading of cervical mucus
   C. Mucus secretion of the cervix
   D. Thinning of the cervical mucus
   E. None of the above
   Ref. 8 - p. 635

4. Intestinal obstruction in a newborn with cystic fibrosis is often due to:
   A. Duodenal atresia
   B. Intussusception
   C. Meconium ileus
   D. Imperforate anus
   E. Intestinal malrotation
   Ref. 4 - p. 1177

5. Cystosarcoma phylloides:
   A. Is a small inconspicuous tumor
   B. Behaves as a malignant tumor from the onset
   C. Arises from an intracanalicular fibroadenoma
   D. Spread is by local invasion
   E. Treatment is by simple mastectomy
   Ref. 6 - p. 540

6. Excessive loss of sodium in the adrenal insufficiency state accounts for:
   A. Increased extra-cellular water
   B. Decreased hematocrit reading
   C. Dilution of plasma protein
   D. Hypovolemia
   E. Lessened blood viscosity
   Ref. 6 - p. 1403

7. A 48-hour-old infant exhibits a scattered rash consisting of papules measuring 3 to 4 mm. with mild erythema and topped with vesicles; the rash looks like "fleabite dermatitis"; the infant is in good health. The rash is most likely:
   A. Erythema toxicum
   B. Lanugo
   C. Milia
   D. Staph. pustules
   E. Cutaneous moniliasis
   Ref. 10 - p. 78

8. The nidus of infection in septic abortion:
   A. Cannot be adequately treated with antibiotics
   B. Should be treated by D & C
   C. Should be treated by hysterectomy at times
   D. All of the above
   E. None of the above   Ref. 9 - pp. 174-176

9. Jaundice in the pediatric age group may be caused by any of the following, except:
   A. Biliary atresia   D. Carcinoma of the pancreas
   B. Choledochal cyst   E. Primary hepatic metabolic
   C. Physiological jaundice   disorder
                                 Ref. 4 - p. 1188

10. Asherman's syndrome may be detected by:
    A. Speculum examination of the cervix
    B. Flat plate of the pelvis
    C. Hysterogram
    D. Culdoscopy
    E. Colposcopy   Ref. 9 - p. 603

11. Acute gastric dilatation may follow:
    A. Serious infection, as pneumonia
    B. Application of hyperextension body cast
    C. Renal stone or infection
    D. Major abdominal operation
    E. Any of the above   Ref. 6 - p. 1077

12. The most common cause of secondary amenorrhea is:
    A. Radiation   D. Refractory uterus
    B. Pelvic inflammatory disease   E. Prolonged progestational
    C. Ovarian failure   intake
                                Ref. 8 - p. 650

13. Precipitating causes of amniotic fluid embolism include:
    A. Prolonged labor   D. Tumultuous labor
    B. Borderline pelvis   E. None of the above
    C. Megaloblastic anemia   Ref. 7 - p. 950

14. The hemorrhage associated with amniotic fluid embolization is related to _____ .
    A. Uterine rupture   D. All
    B. Uterine atony   E. None
    C. Hypofibrinogenemia   Ref. 7 - p. 951

15. The most important toxic manifestation of ethambutol is usually:
    A. Skin rash   D. Jaundice
    B. Epigastric pain   E. Urinary retention
    C. Loss of vision   Ref. 1 - p. 868

16. All of the following statements about herpes zoster are true except:
    A. Second attacks rarely occur
    B. The virus may be cultured from the vesicular fluid
    C. Motor weakness may occur
    D. Cranial nerve involvement is common
    E. Elderly people are affected most often
                                        Ref. 2 - pp. 685-686

17. Chiari-Frommel syndrome:
    A. Lactation continues because of continued lactogenic hormone
    B. Ovarian activity is suspended due to cessation
    C. The underlying cause is usually an emotional disturbance
    D. All of the above
    E. None of the above   Ref. 9 - p. 512

18. The most common agent involved in viral meningitis is:
    A. Measles   D. Adenoviruses
    B. Enteroviruses   E. Influenza
    C. Herpes   Ref. 2 - p. 687

19. Distant metastases from breast cancer are especially frequent because:
    A. Lymph flow is free between the two breasts
    B. Many breast lymphatics empty directly into central veins
    C. The axilla contains many lymph nodes
    D. The breast is highly vascular
    E. Breast cancer is especially malignant
                                        Ref. 6 - p. 529

20. The most common cause of peripheral neuritis in pregnancy is:
    A. Toxicity   D. Iatrogenic
    B. Nutritional   E. Pressure
    C. Trauma   Ref. 9 - p. 295

21. Irregular shedding of the endometrium is due to:
    A. Excess estrogen production
    B. Endometrial failure
    C. Failure of ovulation
    D. Decreased estrogen production
    E. Retarded regression of corpus luteum
                                        Ref. 8 - pp. 79-86, 640

22. Primaquine-sensitive hemolytic anemia is due to the deficiency of:
    A. Phosphoglycerate kinase
    B. Triosephosphate isomerase
    C. Glucose 6-phosphate dehydrogenase
    D. Pyruvate kinase
    E. None of the above   Ref. 1 - p. 1609

23. Oophorectomy at the time of mastectomy for carcinoma of the breast increases the survival rate if:
    A. Patient is pre-menopausal
    B. Patient is post-menopausal
    C. Patient had first pregnancy before age 18
    D. Patient has never been pregnant
    E. Has no effect on survival rate in any case
                                            Ref. 4 - p. 601

24. Hypervolemia in a newborn is associated with:
    A. Stripping of the umbilical cord
    B. Erythroblastosis
    C. Transfused twin in a twin-to-twin transfusion syndrome
    D. All of the above
    E. None of the above   Ref. 10 - p. 97

25. All of the following are correct concerning infant feeding, except:
    A. Gavage feeding is safest for infants below 1650 g at birth
    B. Low-birth weight infants usually have a deficit of mineral stores
    C. Immature infants are unable to digest milk protein
    D. Low-birth weight infants have a decreased ability to absorb cow's milk fat
    E. All newborn babies are able to digest and absorb carbohydrates well   Ref. 10 - pp. 108-110

26. The mean level of estriol excreted in 24 hours at term is:
    A. 25 mg   D. 150 mg
    B. 50 mg   E. 200 mg
    C. 100 mg   Ref. 9 - p. 123

27. Niacin deficiency (pellagra) is usually first manifested by:
    A. Convulsions and coma
    B. Cutaneous lesions
    C. Diplopia
    D. Hyperkinesis, irritability and restlessness
    E. Tremors and loss of fine motor coordination
                                            Ref. 10 - p. 181

28. The most serious contraindication to digital commissurotomy for mitral stenosis is:
    A. Resulting insufficiency cannot be determined
    B. Presence of pulmonary congestion
    C. Extensive calcification of the valve leaflets
    D. Ventricular hypertrophy
    E. Increased left atrial pressure   Ref. 4 - p. 2055

29. The most important source of blood supply to the femoral head is:
    A. Through the ligamentum teres
    B. From the capitellum

C. Medullary vessels of the neck
D. Through visceral capsular vessels
E. From the greater trochanter   Ref. 6 - p. 1819

30. Proper treatment for enchondroma is:
    A. Curettement and bone chip filling
    B. Irradiation therapy
    C. Subperiosteal resection
    D. Amputation
    E. Prolonged immobilization   Ref. 6 - p. 1776

31. Regarding carpal navicular fracture, which is false?
    A. Nonunion is common
    B. The hairline fracture is seen readily on X-ray
    C. Pain is over the snuff-box area
    D. Prolonged immobilization should be tried
    E. Fragment excision is the last resort
                                         Ref. 6 - p. 1816

32. The manifestations of staphylococcal infections may include:
    A. Osteomyelitis
    B. Recurrent folliculitis of the beard area
    C. Involvement of the axillary sweat glands
    D. Carbuncles of the skin
    E. All of the above   Ref. 1 - p. 774

33. Which one of the following statements is true of acute bacterial
    endocarditis?
    A. Normal valves are often involved
    B. Chills are very rare
    C. Osler's nodes are very common
    D. Metastatic abscesses are very rare following septic emboli
    E. It is usually caused by streptococcus viridans
                                         Ref. 1 - p. 763

34. The most successful palliative operation for transposition of
    great vessels is:
    A. Subclavian-aortic anastomosis
    B. Pulmonary artery banding
    C. Aortic-pulmonary window
    D. Creation of atrial septal defect
    E. Closure of patent ductus arteriosus
                                         Ref. 6 - p. 729

35. In severe burns, the fluid requirements after 48 hours are:
    A. Predominantly water to maintain serum Na at 135 mEq/L
    B. Potassium of 60-120 mEq/day
    C. Whole blood to maintain hematocrit at 40 vol/% or above
    D. Total volume to keep adequate urinary excretion and avoid
       pulmonary edema
    E. All of the above   Ref. 6 - p. 262

36. In transposition of great vessels, which statement is false?
    A. Systemic venous flow from right ventricle goes to aorta
    B. Oxygenated blood from left ventricle is returned to aorta
    C. Associated patent ductus is incompatible with life
    D. Associated ventricular septal defect is life saving
    E. Persistent patent foramen ovale is life saving
    Ref. 6 - p. 728

37. Aplastic anemia may occur due to the administration of:
    A. Penicillin   D. Prednisone
    B. Tetracycline   E. None of the above
    C. Chloramphenicol   Ref. 1 - p. 1628

38. The most reliable diagnostic method in bladder rupture is:
    A. Catheterization   D. Await signs of peritoneal
    B. Recovery of injected fluid   irritation
    C. Cystoscopy   E. Retrograde cystogram
    Ref. 4 - p. 1527

39. Diabetes mellitus in young people is characterized by all of the
    following, except:
    A. Polyuria, polyphagia and polydipsia
    B. Nocturia
    C. Weight gain
    D. Fatigability and lethargy
    E. Abdominal pain and vomiting   Ref. 10 - p. 346

40. Adrenocortical insufficiency is characterized by:
    A. Urinary loss of sodium and chloride ions
    B. Excessive water loss
    C. Hemoconcentration
    D. Lowering of blood pressure
    E. All of the above   Ref. 6 - p. 1402

41. A macrocytic peripheral blood smear may be commonly observed
    in:
    A. Celiac disease   D. All of the above
    B. Amethopterin therapy   E. None of the above
    C. Orotic aciduria   Ref. 1 - p. 1586

42. The CSF in a patient with viral meningitis caused by mumps:
    A. Has cloudy fluid and very high protein content
    B. Has early lymphocytosis followed by an increase in neutro-
       phils
    C. Has a glucose content which may be less than 40
    D. All of the above
    E. None of the above   Ref. 2 - p. 689

43. A common cause of total anuria is:
    A. Bilateral cortical necrosis
    B. Nephrotic syndrome
    C. Chronic pyelonephritis
    D. Benign hypertension
    E. None of the above
       Ref. 2 - p. 1108

44. In which way does pregnancy affect Hodgkin's disease?
    A. Unpredictable
    B. No adverse effect on longevity
    C. Exacerbations in the postpartum period
    D. All of the above
    E. None of the above
       Ref. 7 - p. 777

45. Persistent or recurrent talipes equinovarus may require:
    A. Achilles tendon lengthening
    B. Transfer of tibialis anticus tendon to cuboid bone
    C. Wedged plaster cast
    D. Wedge resections and triple arthrodesis
    E. All of the above
       Ref. 6 - p. 1734

46. A cytomegalovirus infection in an immunosuppressed individual
    might lead to:
    A. Hepatitis
    B. Pericarditis
    C. Hemolytic anemia
    D. All of the above
    E. None of the above
       Ref. 2 - p. 696

47. A disease producing abdominal pain similar to that of biliary
    colic can be diagnosed by means of the:
    A. Urinary FIGLU
    B. Ehrlich aldehyde test
    C. Urinary 5 - HIAA
    D. Ferric chloride test
    E. Regitine test
       Ref. 2 - p. 1874

48. The most extreme degree of failure of uterine fusion is:
    A. Uterus subseptus
    B. Uterus unicornis
    C. Uterus bicornis unicollis
    D. Uterus duplex bicornis
    E. Uterus didelphys
       Ref. 8 - pp. 159-163

49. If urine escapes when a patient rises after completion of urina-
    tion, which of the following should be strongly considered?
    A. Bladder infection
    B. Stress incontinence
    C. Urge incontinence
    D. Urethral diverticulum
    E. Neurogenic bladder
       Ref. 8 - pp. 209-210

50. Scalene fat pad biopsy obtains nodes from:
    A. Deep cervical chain
    B. Jugular chain
    C. Carotid sheath chain
    D. Superior mediastinum
    E. Supraclavicular area
       Ref. 6 - pp. 649-650

51. Severely depleted patients with known or suspected malignancies should have an attempt at preoperative restoration of positive nitrogen balance for:
    A. 1-2 days   D. 3-4 weeks
    B. 4-5 days   E. 4-8 weeks
    C. 7-10 days   Ref. 4 - p. 155

52. The least common dermatological disorder of the vulva is:
    A. Seborrhea   D. Herpes
    B. Psoriasis   E. Intertrigo
    C. Folliculitis   Ref. 8 - p. 183

53. Metachromatic leucodystrophy is characterized by all of the following, except:
    A. Disease usually evident during first week of life
    B. Weakness, swallowing difficulties, ataxia and paralysis
    C. Sulfatide accumulates in brain, kidney and bile ducts
    D. No specific treatment
    E. Enzyme defect is a deficiency of enzyme which catalyzes cleavage of sulfuric acid from sulfatide
                                      Ref. 10 - p. 384

54. With regard to the malignant behavior of leiomyosarcomas, the most important criterion is:
    A. Blood vessel penetration by tumor cells
    B. Tumor cells in lymphatic channels
    C. Lymphocyte infiltration
    D. The number of mitoses/high power field
    E. Cellular atypism   Ref. 8 - p. 386

55. Anticholinesterases may constitute an important adjunct to the management of alveolar hypoventilation in patients with:
    A. Amyotrophic lateral sclerosis D. Guillain-Barré syndrome
    B. Myasthenia gravis   E. Progressive muscular
    C. Poliomyelitis   dystrophy
                                      Ref. 2 - p. 804

56. The manifestations of primary tuberculosis may include:
    A. Pleurisy with effusion   D. Meningitis
    B. Cervical lymphadenitis   E. All of the above
    C. Miliary tuberculosis   Ref. 1 - p. 860

57. Sarcoidosis producing asymptomatic hilar adenopathy without pulmonary parenchymal disease usually requires:
    A. Adrenal steroid therapy   D. Colchicine therapy
    B. No therapy   E. Chloroquine therapy
    C. Oxyphenbutasone therapy   Ref. 1 - p. 1062

58. Treatment of acute renal failure includes which of the following?
   A. Reduction in toxic split protein products in the blood
   B. Correction of acidosis and hyponatremia
   C. Prevention or correction of hyperkalemia
   D. Prevention of fluid overload
   E. All of the above   Ref. 6 - p. 1565

59. A major underlying factor in cardiac arrest or ventricular fibrillation is:
   A. Muscle infarction
   B. Vessel thrombosis
   C. Conduction failure
   D. Anoxia
   E. Chemical toxic effect
        Ref. 6 - p. 759

60. Hepatic granulomas may be produced by:
   A. Sarcoidosis
   B. Tuberculosis
   C. Brucellosis
   D. Beryllium poisoning
   E. All of the above
        Ref. 2 - p. 1352

61. The most sensitive test of liver function is probably the:
   A. SGOT
   B. BSP clearance
   C. Prothrombin time
   D. Serum albumin concentration
   E. Alkaline phosphatase
        Ref. 2 - p. 1332

62. The complications of acute myocardial infarction may include:
   A. Ventricular arrhythmias
   B. Shock
   C. Pulmonary edema
   D. All of the above
   E. None of the above
        Ref. 1 - pp. 1205-1206

63. IgM is of greater molecular weight than:
   A. IgG
   B. IgD
   C. IgA serum
   D. All of the above
   E. None of the above
        Ref. 10 - p. 433

64. Distal femoral epiphyses are not often seen before:
   A. 32 weeks
   B. 34 weeks
   C. 35 weeks
   D. 37 weeks
   E. 40 weeks
        Ref. 7 - pp. 200-204

65. Initiation of lactation is caused by:
   A. Posterior pituitary release of prolactin
   B. Anterior pituitary release of prolactin
   C. Oxytocic effect
   D. None of the above
   E. B and C   Ref. 7 - p. 470

66. Renal papillary necrosis may result most commonly from the ingestion of:
   A. Penicillin
   B. Phenacetin
   C. Cortisone
   D. Allopurinol
   E. Antihistamines
        Ref. 2 - p. 1147

67. Which one of the following statements regarding pulmonary tuberculosis due to Battey bacillus is true?
A. The infection usually resolves without treatment
B. It is a photochromogen
C. An excellent therapeutic response to INH and streptomycin may be expected
D. It is a nonchromogene
E. The bacillus characteristically produces nicotinic acid on culture Ref. 1 - p. 874

68. Which of the following chemotherapeutic agents, when given systemically, inhibits cell division in wounds:
A. Nitrogen mustard D. All of the above
B. Thio-TEPA E. None of the above
C. 5-fluorouracil Ref. 4 - p. 266

69. Carcinoid syndrome usually does not occur unless there are metastases to:
A. Liver D. Skin
B. Lung E. Bone
C. Brain Ref. 6 - p. 1098

70. Forced diuresis together with high intake of sodium chloride is recommended in treating intoxication due to:
A. Barbiturates D. Bromide
B. Phenothiazines E. Lead
C. Arsenic Ref. 2 - p. 592

71. Of the following vasoactive drugs, the one most useful in the treatment of septic shock is:
A. Levarterenol D. Norepinephrine
B. Metaraminol E. Neosynephrine
C. Isoproterenol Ref. 1 - p. 738

72. The manifestations of disseminated tuberculosis may include:
A. Anemia D. All of the above
B. Low grade fever E. None of the above
C. Splenomegaly Ref. 1 - p. 865

73. Placental insufficiency is most frequently seen in:
A. Erythroblastosis fetalis D. Oligohydramnios
B. Toxemia E. Placenta previa
C. Hydramnios Ref. 7 - pp. 590-592

74. An acute episode of asthma, causing obvious distress, can be treated with _____ of a 1:1,000 concentration of aqueous epinephrine hydrochloride by subcutaneous injection:
A. 0.005 to 0.008 ml D. 0.5 to 1.0 ml
B. 0.05 to 0.2 ml E. 1.5 to 2.5 ml
C. 0.30 to 0.5 ml Ref. 10 - p. 466

75. Parasitic infections which can cause urticaria:
    A. Ascaris
    B. Strongyloides
    C. Amebae
    D. All of the above
    E. None of the above
    Ref. 10 - p. 477

76. Brain tumors manifest themselves by which mechanism?
    A. Compression of neural tissue
    B. Invasion and destruction of neural tissue
    C. Alteration of blood supply
    D. Alteration of cerebrospinal fluid circulation
    E. All of the above
    Ref. 6 - p. 1647

77. Glucagon:
    A. Accelerates incorporation of amino acids into liver protein
    B. Stimulates hepatic glycogenolysis
    C. Inhibits gluconeogenesis in liver
    D. Inhibits lipolysis in adipose tissue
    E. Inhibits secretion of insulin from B cells of the pancreas
    Ref. 1 - p. 560

78. A five-year-old with streptococcal pharyngitis is best treated
    with:
    A. Erythromycin, 250 mg, qid, po
    B. Penicillin, 200,000 units, qid, po
    C. 600,000 units of procaine penicillin, I.M., for 10 days
    D. Chloramphenicol 250 mg, qid, po
    E. 600,000 units of benzathine penicillin, I.M.
    Ref. 10 - p. 502

79. The most common cause of renal failure in patients presenting
    for dialysis and transplantation usually is:
    A. Chronic glomerulonephritis
    B. Acute pyelonephritis
    C. Ureteral calculus
    D. Lipoid nephrosis
    E. Polyarteritis nodosa
    Ref. 2 - p. 1124

80. Curling's ulcer is a major complication of burns, with an in-
    cidence of ____ per cent, a peak incidence in the first ____ hours;
    it is usually found in the:
    A. 25 to 45; 48; duodenum
    B. 15 to 35; 24; stomach
    C. 10 to 25; 72; gastroduodenal area
    D. 5 to 15; 48; jejunum
    E. 10 to 15; 96; ileum
    Ref. 10 - p. 523

81. The most ominous kind of pain with peripheral vascular disease
    is:
    A. Rest pain, usually due to tissue necrosis and ischemic
       neuritis
    B. Intermittent muscle pain due to arterial spasm
    C. Abrupt, constant pain with arterial occlusion
    D. Burning type pain with skin ulceration
    E. Numb type of pain with digital gangrene
    Ref. 6 - p. 841

82. Reduction of the flea population may be useful in the control of:
   A. Rocky Mountain spotted fever
   B. Rickettsialpox
   C. Murine typhus
   D. Q fever
   E. None of the above
   Ref. 2 - p. 254

83. In patients with neoplastic obstruction of the common bile duct:
   A. The gallbladder is never distended
   B. The gallbladder is rarely distended
   C. The gallbladder is frequently distended
   D. Tenderness is rarely present
   E. The prognosis is generally excellent
   Ref. 2 - p. 1322

84. Regarding traction diverticulum of the esophagus:
   A. Most common through cricopharyngeus muscle
   B. Contains all elements of the esophageal wall
   C. Filling of sac obstructs the esophageal lumen
   D. May ulcerate from retained, decomposed food
   E. Apt to rupture from over-distention
   Ref. 6 - p. 1023

85. Mites are the reservoir of which of the following rickettsial diseases?
   A. Q fever
   B. Murine typhus
   C. Rocky Mountain spotted fever
   D. Rickettsialpox
   E. None of the above
   Ref. 2 - p. 258

86. The following physical finding may be useful in making the diagnosis of angina pectoris in patients during an attack:
   A. A loud first heart sound
   B. A loud second heart sound
   C. The presence of a fourth heart sound
   D. An opening snap
   E. None of the above
   Ref. 1 - p. 1195

87. Which method yields the best results in the treatment of Bartholin abscess?
   A. Aspiration
   B. Incision and drainage
   C. Primary excision
   D. Marsupialization
   E. Heat and antibiotics
   Ref. 9 - p. 596

88. Which one of the following is generally not a feature of Felty's syndrome?
   A. Rheumatoid arthritis
   B. Splenomegaly
   C. Polycythemia
   D. Granulocytopenia
   E. Lymphadenopathy
   Ref. 2 - p. 149

89. Thyrotoxic crisis may require treatment with:
   A. Digitalis
   B. Propylthiouracil
   C. Intravenous iodine
   D. All of the above
   E. None of the above
   Ref. 1 - p. 481

90. Treatment of cervical pregnancy is:
   A. Allow to progress to term   D. Hysterectomy
   B. D & C   E. Excision of cervix
   C. Simple excision   Ref. 7 - p. 561

91. Bilateral symmetrical renal cortical necrosis is seen most frequently due to:
   A. Toxemia   D. Amniotic fluid embolism
   B. Septic abortion   E. Mismatched blood
   C. Abruptio placenta   Ref. 9 - p. 569

92. Which one of the following is under anterior pituitary control?
   A. Gonad function in male and female
   B. Growth of young animals
   C. Control of blood pressure
   D. Muscle activity
   E. Fluid and electrolyte balance   Ref. 6 - p. 1365

93. The basic attempt in repair of urinary stress incontinence is to:
   A. Lengthen urethra to normal and prevent its collapse in erect position
   B. Tighten urethral sphincter
   C. Put muscle sling under urethra
   D. Decrease bladder tone
   E. Give muscle exercise program   Ref. 4 - p. 1478

94. The normal serum concentration range of folic acid assayed microbiologically is approximately:
   A. 5 to 20 ng/ml   D. 5-10 mg/ml
   B. 1 to 4 mg/ml   E. 50-100 mg/ml
   C. 1 to 4 ng/ml   Ref. 1 - p. 1589

95. In "warm" septic shock, the cardiac index is:
   A. Increased   D. Variable
   B. Decreased   E. Unknown
   C. Unchanged   Ref. 4 - p. 81

96. Significant penetrating wounds of the neck should be explored only if:
   A. There is subcutaneous emphysema
   B. There is uncontrollable bleeding
   C. There is upper respiratory distress
   D. The wound is anterior to the sternocleidomastoid
   E. In all cases   Ref. 4 - p. 367

97. At about the time of the first missed menstrual period, detection of which of the following constitutes a positive pregnancy test?
   A. Luteinizing hormone (LH)
   B. Human chorionic gonadotropin (HCG)
   C. Follicle stimulating hormone (FSH)
   D. Luteotropic hormone (LTH)
   E. Progesterone   Ref. 6 - p. 1593

98. Spinal puncture should be used to determine:
    A. Spinal fluid pressure
    B. Whether a block exists
    C. Types and numbers of cells present
    D. Protein and sugar levels
    E. All of the above   Ref. 6 - p. 1637

99. In pectus excavatum:
    A. The manubrium is markedly depressed
    B. The xiphoid is elevated and prominent
    C. The heart is in dextro-position
    D. The rib cartilages are elongated
    E. Cardiac pressure is the main reason for repair
                                  Ref. 6 - p. 602

100. In pregnancy, peripheral resistance to insulin utilization is
     caused by:
     A. Chorionic somatomammotropin
     B. Estrogen
     C. Progesterone
     D. None of the above
     E. All of the above   Ref. 7 - p. 791

101. The factor not associated with any increase in the incidence of
     ischemic heart disease is:
     A. Diabetes mellitus   D. Hyperlipemia
     B. Hypertension   E. None of the above
     C. Excessive smoking   Ref. 1 - p. 1194

102. Class B pregnant diabetics should be admitted to the hospital
     for evaluation for delivery no later than:
     A. 32 weeks   D. 38 weeks
     B. 34 weeks   E. 40 weeks
     C. 36 weeks   Ref. 7 - p. 795

103. Which of the following is not an indication for operation in
     nodular nontoxic goiter?
     A. Esophageal or tracheal obstruction
     B. Development of toxic goiter
     C. Danger of development of thyroiditis
     D. Danger of carcinomatous degeneration
     E. Cosmetic factors   Ref. 6 - p. 1448

104. A prolonged latent phase in labor is associated with:
     A. An unripe cervix
     B. Early analgesia with sedation
     C. Early use of conduction anesthesic
     D. All of the above
     E. None of the above   Ref. 7 - p. 838

105. The infections occurring during organ transplantation and fol-
low-up immunosuppressive therapy with azathioprine and corti-
costeroids frequently include:
   A. Staphylococcal infections
   B. Cytomegalovirus infections
   C. Pneumocystis carinii infections
   D. Monilia infections
   E. All of the above   Ref. 1 - p. 733

106. Which statement regarding malignant synovioma is false?
   A. Most common in the knee
   B. Highly sensitive to X-ray therapy
   C. Lung metastasis after attempted resection is frequent
   D. Treatment results are highly unsatisfactory
   E. Neither radical resection nor amputation is successful
                                          Ref. 4 - p. 1397

107. BAL, EDTA and penicillamine may be used in treating poison-
ing with:
   A. Lead   D. Copper
   B. Arsenic   E. All of the above
   C. Mercury   Ref. 10 - p. 534

108. Ascites and hydrothorax are associated with:
   A. Struma ovarii   D. Krukenberg tumor of ovary
   B. Fibroma of ovary   E. None of the above
   C. Theca-luteum cyst of ovary   Ref. 8 - p. 471

109. Roentgenograms revealing metaphyseal fragmentation, perios-
teal hemorrhages with calcification, squaring of long bones
due to new bone formation and multiple fractures are most
strongly suggestive of:
   A. Osteogenesis imperfecta   D. Child abuse
   B. 18-Trisomy syndrome   E. Metaphyseal dysostosis
   C. Chondroectodermal dysplasia   Ref. 10 - p. 557

110. Causes of hirsutism in women commonly include:
   A. Familial trait   D. Congenital adrenal hyper-
   B. Polycystic ovaries   plasia
   C. Adrenal carcinoma   E. All of the above
                                 Ref. 1 - pp. 286, 512

111. Treatment of early esophageal perforations consists of:
   A. Left tube thoracostomy
   B. Right tube thoracostomy
   C. Thoracotomy and drainage
   D. Thoracotomy, direct suture and drainage
   E. Thoracotomy and direct suture, no drainage
                                 Ref. 4 - p. 379

112. Bullet wounds near major blood vessels should be explored only if:
    A. There is no pulse
    B. The pulse is weakened
    C. The extremity is cold
    D. The fingers or toes are paralyzed
    E. In all cases, regardless of physical findings
    Ref. 4 - p. 387

113. The principal cause of death in renal transplant recipients is:
    A. Rejection
    B. Infection
    C. Uremia
    D. Malignancy
    E. Hemorrhage
    Ref. 4 - p. 465

114. The perinatal period is:
    A. The week before and the week after delivery
    B. The period of gestation after the 20th week through the 27th day after birth
    C. From the 28th week of gestation through the first seven days after birth
    D. From conception to 28 days after birth
    E. "Around the time of birth"
    Ref. 9 - p. 4

115. Embryological primordial egg cells are called:
    A. Waldeyer cords
    B. Mayer's patches
    C. Kopferer cords
    D. Warthin's cords
    E. Strauss' patches
    Ref. 8 - p. 126

116. Concerning withdrawal symptoms from short-acting barbiturate or glutethimide:
    A. Symptoms first appear 48 to 72 hours later
    B. Initial symptoms are convulsions and coma
    C. Gradual withdrawal under medical supervision recommended
    D. All of the above
    E. None of the above
    Ref. 10 - p. 564

117. Probably the most successful operation for breast cancer is:
    A. Radical mastectomy with internal mammary dissection
    B. Radical mastectomy with supraclavicular dissection
    C. Radical mastectomy with removal of breast, pectoral muscles and axillary tissue
    D. Simple mastectomy and irradiation
    E. Radical mastectomy sparing the pectoral muscles
    Ref. 6 - p. 541

118. Myocardial rupture as a complication of myocardial infarction is most likely to occur during the:
    A. First week
    B. Second week
    C. Third week
    D. Fourth week
    E. None of the above
    Ref. 1 - p. 1209

119. Chronic Hashimoto's thyroiditis presents as:
   A. Hyperthyroidism   D. Mass in the neck
   B. Hypothyroidism   E. Carcinoma of the thyroid
   C. Tracheal obstruction   Ref. 4 - p. 629

120. A child is diagnosed as having meningitis due to Haemophilus
   influenzae; he should receive as initial treatment:
   A. Ampicillin 150 mg/kg, IV in 30 minutes in saline solution,
      3 ml/100 mg of drug
   B. Kanamycin 7.5 mg, I.M.
   C. Sodium penicillin G, 1,200,000 units IV in 30 minutes in
      50 ml/m^2 of saline
   D. Chloramphenicol succinate 50 mg/kg in 3-4 ml of saline
      over 30 minutes
   E. All of the above   Ref. 10 - p. 603

121. Transient foot drop in the postpartum period after a spontaneous
   delivery may be due to:
   A. Hysteria   D. Sciatic nerve damage
   B. Lumbosacral damage   E. Peroneal nerve damage
   C. Tibial nerve damage   Ref. 9 - p. 295

122. Mee's lines in the finger nails are an important diagnostic
   feature of chronic _____ poisoning:
   A. Mercury   D. Beryllium
   B. Lead   E. Manganese
   C. Arsenic   Ref. 2 - p. 58

123. All of the following are characteristic of parapertussis, except:
   A. An acute infection of respiratory tract
   B. No cross immunity with pertussis and parapertussis
   C. Incubation period approximately 7 to 14 days
   D. Course of disease often ends within 2 or 3 weeks
   E. Complications include pneumonia and myocarditis
                                    Ref. 10 - p. 632

124. The mortality from staphylococcal food poisoning is:
   A. 5%   D. 14%
   B. 8%   E. None of the above
   C. 10%   Ref. 10 - p. 647

125. Acute obstruction of the colon is more of a surgical emergency
   than obstruction of the small bowel because:
   A. The colon can hold a greater volume of fluid and gas
   B. Colon bacteria are more numerous and virulent
   C. The competent ileocecal valve makes a closed loop
   D. The diagnosis is more easily made
   E. Strangulation is more frequent   Ref. 6 - p. 987

126. _____ % of thyroid nodules "cold" to I^{131} are malignant.
    A. 10-20%   D. 70-80%
    B. 20-30%   E. 80-90%
    C. 50-60%   Ref. 4 - p. 644

127. By the seventh postnatal year there are _____ oocytes:
    A. 600,000   D. 2,000
    B. 300,000   E. None of the above
    C. 1,000,000   Ref. 8 - p. 130

128. Common features of hereditary spherocytosis include:
    A. Jaundice and splenomegaly
    B. Mild anemia
    C. Chronic leg ulcers
    D. Hemolysis beginning in vitro at about 0.64% saline solution
    E. All of the above   Ref. 1 - p. 1608

129. Which of the following is not characteristic of acute gastric dilatation:
    A. Crampy, colicky pain
    B. Almost continuous overflow vomiting
    C. Hiccup often present and persistent
    D. Prostration and hypovolemic shock are severe
    E. Upper abdomen is distended and dull
                                   Ref. 6 - p. 1077

130. The most common presenting clinical finding of hyperparathyroidism is:
    A. Pathologic fracture   D. Duodenal ulcer
    B. Renal failure   E. Pancreatitis
    C. Nephrolithiasis   Ref. 4 - p. 661

131. In the majority of cases, primary tuberculosis is characterized by:
    A. Fevers, spiking to 102 degrees
    B. Anorexia, lethargy and weight loss
    C. Paroxysmal cough and chest pain
    D. All of the above
    E. None of the above   Ref. 10 - p. 665

132. Hydrocephaly is most commonly associated with:
    A. Spina bifida   D. All of the above
    B. Breech presentation   E. A and B only
    C. Erythroblastosis   Ref. 7 - p. 885

133. Induced emesis in a conscious patient is usually contraindicated if poisoning occurred with the ingestion of:
    A. Phenobarbital   D. Lye
    B. Antihistamines   E. Darvon
    C. Amphetamines   Ref. 2 - p. 57

134. Features of the Pickwickian syndrome may include:
    A. Obesity   D. Hypercapnia
    B. Somnolence   E. All of the above
    C. Polycythemia   Ref. 2 - p. 1378

135. Achalasia in children is best treated by:
    A. Observation   D. Esophagomyotomy
    B. Muscle relaxant   E. Distal esophagectomy and
    C. Dilatation   primary anastamosis
                                       Ref. 4 - p. 726

136. In severe hypospadias, the possibility of an intersex problem
    is settled by:
    A. Careful inspection of genitals
    B. Biopsy for gonadal tissue
    C. Karyotyping
    D. Hormone assay
    E. Laparotomy   Ref. 6 - p. 1571

137. An increased number of white blood cells in the urinary sedi-
    ment unaccompanied by any other cellular elements usually is
    most suggestive of:
    A. Chronic glomerulonephritis D. Chronic pyelonephritis
    B. Malignant hypertension   E. Thrombotic thrombocyto-
    C. Lupus nephritis   penic purpura
                                       Ref. 2 - p. 1150

138. Characteristic features of anaplastic carcinoma of the thyroid
    include:
    A. Appearance in adolescence
    B. Excellent response to radiotherapy
    C. Low order of malignancy
    D. All of the above
    E. None of the above   Ref. 1 - p. 482

139. A characteristic laboratory finding in infectious mononucleosis
    is:
    A. Hemolytic anemia
    B. Thrombocytopenia is common
    C. Depressed serum transaminase
    D. Lymphocytic leukocytosis
    E. All of the above   Ref. 2 - p. 1526

140. In progressive hypopituitarism, of the following the first to
    stop being secreted is:
    A. Thyroid-stimulating hormone
    B. Follicle-stimulating and luteinizing hormone
    C. ACTH
    D. Melanocyte-stimulating hormone
    E. Somatotropic hormone   Ref. 8 - p. 18

141. Lymphocytic choriomeningitis shows a dramatic response to:
    A. Penicillin   D. Methotrexate
    B. Corticosteroids   E. None of the above
    C. Amphotericin B   Ref. 10 - p. 729

142. Characteristic features of subacute thyroiditis often include:
    A. Thyroid tenderness   D. All of the above
    B. Normal RAIU   E. None of the above
    C. A paradoxically low ESR   Ref. 1 - p. 483

143. Patients with diabetic retinopathy are prone to develop a sudden
     temporary loss of vision due to:
    A. Development of glaucoma   D. Hemorrhage into the vit-
    B. Cataract formation   reous
    C. Microaneurysm formation   E. None of the above
                                    Ref. 1 - p. 534

144. The most common cause of postpartum hypopituitarism is:
    A. Thrombophlebitis   D. Eclampsia
    B. Postpartum psychosis   E. Massive hemorrhage
    C. Cerebral hemorrhage   Ref. 8 - p. 663

145. A hypochromic, microcytic anemia with increased iron stores
     in the bone marrow may be:
    A. Iron responsive   D. Pyridoxine responsive
    B. Vitamin B_{12} responsive   E. Ascorbic acid responsive
    C. Vitamin A responsive   Ref. 1 - p. 1584

146. The incidence of gallstones in American Indians is:
    A. Greatly increased
    B. Greatly decreased
    C. Equal to that of the general population
    D. Decreased in females only
    E. Decreased in young males   Ref. 2 - p. 1309

147. The causative mechanism of post-stenotic vascular dilatation
     is:
    A. Jet impingement   D. Reduced vis-a-tergo
    B. Swirl effect of blood   E. Venturi effect
    C. Lateral stagnation of flow   Ref. 6 - p. 696

148. The nerve injured by fracture or callus healing of the humeral
     medial condyle is:
    A. Radial   D. Musculocutaneous
    B. Median   E. Lesser sural
    C. Ulnar   Ref. 4 - p. 1341

149. The most common type of esophageal hiatus hernia is:
    A. Paraesophageal   D. Morgagni
    B. Sliding type   E. None of the above
    C. Bochdalek   Ref. 4 - p. 745

150. Rubella is characterized by all of the following, except:
A. Worldwide distribution
B. Generalized maculopapular rash and postauricular lympha-
denopathy
C. Major complications include otitis media and pneumonia
D. Epidemics occurred in USA in approximately 6 to 9 year
intervals
E. Serological studies reveal that 75 to 90% of adult Americans
have had rubella in the past   Ref. 10 - pp. 759-760

151. The Australia antigen has been observed in serum from patients
with:
A. Crigler-Najjar syndrome   D. Carcinoma of the colon
B. Infectious mononucleosis   E. Familial polyposis
C. Hepatitis   Ref. 2 - p. 1335

152. Pyloric channel ulcers are considered to be:
A. Gastric ulcers in behavior   D. A form of gastritis
B. Duodenal ulcers in behavior   E. None of the above
C. Malignant ulcers   Ref. 4 - p. 830

153. Virtually all fetal heart structures form between _____ weeks
of pregnancy:
A. 3rd to 8th   D. 21st to 26th
B. 9th to 14th   E. 27th to 33rd
C. 15th to 20th   Ref. 6 - p. 677

154. In myocardial infarction which of the following serum enzymes
rises latest and remains elevated for the longest duration?
A. SGOT   D. Aldolase
B. CPK   E. Alkaline phosphatase
C. LDH   Ref. 1 - p. 1200

155. The pressure measured during uterine contractions in the first
stage of labor is:
A. 5 mm Hg   D. 30 mm Hg
B. 10 mm Hg   E. 60 mm Hg
C. 25 mm Hg   Ref. 7 - p. 352

156. The usual cause of perforation in colon cancer is:
A. Tumor slough   D. Volvulus and vascular oc-
B. Tension gangrene   clusion
C. Pressure of impacted feces   E. Intussusception
                                              Ref. 6 - p. 983

157. The most frequent complication of amebiasis is:
A. Lung abscess   D. Hemolytic anemia and bone
B. Liver abscess   marrow suppression
C. Convulsions and coma   E. Retinal dettachment
                                              Ref. 10 - p. 829

158. Fibrinoid deposits in the placental intervillous space at the fetal maternal junction are called:
    A. Hoffbauer's fibrin
    B. Nitabuch's stria
    C. Rohr's stria
    D. Brosen's layer
    E. None of the above
    Ref. 7 - p. 154

159. All of the following may be effective in treating a child with hyperactivity (as part of minimal brain dysfunction syndrome), except:
    A. Dextroamphetamine sulfate
    B. Phenobarbital
    C. Methylphenidate hydrochloride
    D. Thioridazine
    E. Chlorpromazine
    Ref. 10 - pp. 881-882

160. Each of the following parasites commonly invades the liver, except:
    A. Schistosoma mansoni
    B. Clonorchis sinensis
    C. Fasciola hepatica
    D. Echinococcus granulosus
    E. Trichinosis
    Ref. 2 - p. 530

161. Each of the following is a well-recognized complication of ulcerative colitis, except:
    A. Diabetes
    B. Fatty infiltration of the liver
    C. Arthritis
    D. Pyoderma gangrenosum
    E. Erythema nodosum
    Ref. 2 - p. 1271

162. Each of the following measures may be useful in the treatment of paroxysmal atrial tachycardia, except:
    A. Carotid sinus massage
    B. Administration of atropine
    C. Administration of digitalis preparations
    D. Administration of phenylephrine
    E. Administration of prostigmine   Ref. 1 - p. 1133

163. The usual features of chronic granulomatous disease of childhood include all of the following, except:
    A. Recurrent infections with bacteria of low virulence are common
    B. The neutrophils lack the ability to phagocytize bacteria normally
    C. Eczematoid dermatitis is commonly found in these patients
    D. The neutrophils lack the ability to kill the phagocytized bacteria
    E. The morphologic appearance of the neutrophils is normal
    Ref. 1 - p. 320

164. Proteinuria exceeding 3 grams per 24 hours may be commonly found in each of the following, except:
    A. Renal amyloidosis
    B. Obstructive uropathy
    C. Membranous glomerulonephritis
    D. Diabetic nephropathy
    E. Malignant hypertension
    Ref. 2 - p. 1156

165. Which one of the following chromosomal abnormalities is least likely to be associated with mental retardation:
    A. Translocation Down syndrome
    B. Partial deletion of short arm of chromosome No. 5
    C. Turner's syndrome
    D. Klinefelter's syndrome
    E. Trisomy 13   Ref. 10 - p. 888

166. In stress ulcers, the most important diagnostic procedure is:
    A. Arteriography   D. Quantitation of gastric as-
    B. Upper GI series   pirate
    C. Gastroscopy   E. Laparotomy
                                  Ref. 4 - p. 843

167. All of the following are true concerning transverse lie, except:
    A. More common in multiparas than primigravidas
    B. Increased incidence of placenta previa
    C. Seen with pelvic inlet contraction
    D. Usually undergoes spontaneous evolution
    E. Uterine malformations or pelvic tumors may prevent the head or breech from entering the pelvis
                                  Ref. 9 - p. 892

168. All of the following may result in chronic renal failure, except:
    A. Collagen diseases   D. Primary hypoparathyroidism
    B. Obstructive uropathy   E. Polycystic kidney
    C. Glomerulo or pyelonephritis   Ref. 6 - p. 1422

169. The most common cause of colon obstruction is:
    A. Adhesions   D. Neoplasm
    B. Hernias   E. Volvulus
    C. Diverticulitis   Ref. 4 - p. 881

170. Each of the following penicillins is penicillinase-resistant, except:
    A. Methicillin   D. Nafcillin
    B. Ampicillin   E. Cloxacillin
    C. Oxacillin   Ref. 1 - p. 745

171. Each of the following is a common feature of chronic congestive heart failure due to ischemic heart disease, except:
    A. Dyspnea   D. Kerley B lines by X-ray
    B. Basal pulmonary rales   E. Leg edema
    C. Small heart by X-ray   Ref. 1 - p. 1120

172. Common reactions to whole blood transfusions include each of the following, except:
    A. Fever   D. Hypercalcemia
    B. Hemolysis   E. Hypocalcemia
    C. Urticaria   Ref. 1 - pp. 1639-1640

173. With few exceptions, the treatment of small bowel obstruction is:
    A. Surgery
    B. Nasogastric suction
    C. Long intestinal tube (e.g., Miller-Abbott, Cantor)
    D. Enemas
    E. Cathartics   Ref. 4 - p. 886

174. Neuromyelitis optica (Devic's disease) is probably a form of:
    A. Disseminated or multiple sclerosis
    B. Parkinsonism
    C. Hurler's disease
    D. Niemann-Pick disease
    E. Subacute sclerosing panencephalitis
                                     Ref. 10 - p. 918

175. Regarding obstructive congenital cardiovascular lesions, all are correct, except:
    A. They result in systolic overloading
    B. Clinical examination and X-ray films do not show an enlarged heart
    C. Cardiac dilatation is a prominent feature
    D. ECG indicates degree of ventricular hypertrophy
    E. Cardiac failure is late and pre-terminal
                                     Ref. 6 - p. 679

176. Which of the following anesthetic agents may result in extreme uterine relaxation:
    A. Trichlorethylene   D. Cyclopropane
    B. Ether   E. Chloroform
    C. N_2O Ref. 7 - p. 435

177. Hidradenitis suppurativa is found in all regions, except:
    A. Axilla   D. Periumbilical
    B. Circumanal   E. Groin
    C. Scalp   Ref. 4 - p. 1453

178. Hemodialysis is often extremely effective in treating intoxication due to each of the following drugs, except:
    A. Barbital   D. Short-acting barbiturates
    B. Phenobarbital   E. None of the above
    C. Bromide   Ref. 2 - p. 605

179. Each of the following blood clotting factors is synthesized by the liver, except:
    A. Prothrombin   D. Factor IX
    B. Factor V   E. None of the above
    C. Factor VII   Ref. 2 - p. 1330

180. The usual causes of low arterial oxygen tension include each
   of the following, except:
   A. Ventilation-perfusion ratio inequality
   B. Hyperventilation at sea level
   C. Hypoventilation at sea level
   D. Right-to-left shunt
   E. Impaired diffusion across the alveoli
   Ref. 1 - p. 1268

181. Each of the following may occur as a sequel to chronic empy-
   ema, except:
   A. Anemia   D. Weight loss
   B. Malnutrition   E. Secondary amyloidosis
   C. Primary amyloidosis   Ref. 1 - p. 1328

182. Insulin levels in maturity-onset diabetes are usually:
   A. Actually increased   D. Absent
   B. Normal   E. Less than in juvenile dia-
   C. Decreased   betes
                                Ref. 1 - p. 535

183. Each of the following agents may be useful in the treatment of
   lead poisoning, except:
   A. Sodium nitrite   D. Calcium gluconate
   B. EDTA   E. Urea infusion
   C. Penicillamine   Ref. 2 - p. 60

184. Pseudotumor cerebri is frequently associated with:
   A. Convulsions
   B. Increased intracranial pressure
   C. Severe mental retardation
   D. Increased sugar and protein in CSF
   E. Hemiparesis   Ref. 10 - p. 957

185. In young children, the main elements in operative repair of
   pectus excavatum are all of the following, except:
   A. Excision of elongated, depressed costal cartilages
   B. Wedge osteotomy at sterno-manubrial junction
   C. Metal struts to maintain corrected position until healed
   D. Excision of xiphoid process and division of deep attachments
   E. Breakup of retrosternal pericardial attachments
   Ref. 6 - p. 604

186. Brenner tumors of the ovary are associated with:
   A. A high rate of malignancy
   B. Mucinous transformation
   C. "Coffee bean" cells
   D. B and C only
   E. A and B only   Ref. 8 - pp. 472-476

187. Regarding mumps orchitis, all are true, except:
    A. Virus infection accompanying acute parotitis
    B. Estrogens may be helpful
    C. Other steroids are contraindicated because of infection
    D. Incision of tunica albuginea may prevent pressure atrophy
    E. Testicular atrophy is an uncommon sequela
    Ref. 4 - p. 1564

188. An association has been made between the use of phenformin and the development of:
    A. Respiratory acidosis
    B. Metabolic alkalosis
    C. Lactic acidosis
    D. Metabolic acidosis without an anion gap
    E. None of the above
    Ref. 1 - p. 543

Each group of questions below consists of lettered headings followed by a list of numbered words or phrases. For each numbered word or phrase select the one heading which is most closely related to it:

A. Epoophoron
B. Oogonia
C. Rete ovarii
D. Ovarian cortex
E. Interstitial cells

189. ___ Spermatogonia
190. ___ Rete testis
191. ___ Leydig cells
192. ___ Epididymis
193. ___ Tunica vaginalis   Ref. 8 - pp. 130, 528

A. Down syndrome
B. 18-Trisomy
C. 13-Trisomy
D. Cat-Eye syndrome
E. Cri-du-chat syndrome

194. ___ Epicanthal folds, slanting palpebral fissures, microcephaly, round face, mental retardation
195. ___ Hypertelorism, coloboma of iris, preauricular fistula, anal atresia, possible mental retardation
196. ___ Polydactyly, hyperconvex fingernails, hemangiomas, cleft palate and hare-lip, defects of forebrain, mental deficiency
197. ___ Upward slant to palpebral fissures, short hands, clinodactyly, hypotonid, Brushfield spots, mental retardation
198. ___ Microstomia, fish-like mouth, clenched hand, overlapping fingers, short palpebral fissure, short stature, mental retardation   Ref. 11 - pp. 1699-1700

A. Pregnancy
B. Hypothyroidism
C. Hyperthyroidism
D. Chronic liver disease
E. Hashimoto's disease

199. ___ Decrease in thyroxine-binding globulin
200. ___ Increase in thyroxine-binding globulin
201. ___ Prolongation of Achilles reflex time
202. ___ Most patients have antithyroglobulin in the serum
203. ___ Many patients have long-acting thyroid stimulator in the
serum   Ref. 1 - pp. 469-471

Match the following:

A. Carcinoid tumor
B. Adenocarcinoma
C. Both
D. Neither

204. ___ Most common site is rectosigmoid
205. ___ Most common site is appendix
206. ___ Occur anywhere in gastrointestinal tract
207. ___ Hepatic metastases should be resected, if possible
208. ___ Secrete serotonin   Ref. 4 - pp. 908-910

Match the following:

A. Diverticulosis
B. Diverticulitis
C. Both
D. Neither

209. ___ More commonly presents as massive rectal bleeding
210. ___ May be an asymptomatic X-ray finding
211. ___ May cause pneumaturia
212. ___ Has malignant potential
213. ___ May cause obstruction   Ref. 4 - p. 958

A. Oxalates and oxalic acid poisoning
B. Phenolphthalein poisoning
C. Organic phosphorus poisoning
D. Salicylate poisoning
E. Warfarin poisoning

214. ___ Gradual depression of prothrombin levels leading to spontaneous hemorrhages
215. ___ Local irritation, rapid absorption and quick death, com-
bimed with ionized calcium of the blood, heart stops in
diastole, if there is recovery acute renal tubular necrosis
may occur

216. ___ May be found in laxatives, toxic range unknown, cathartic action
217. ___ Anticholinesterase compounds, very toxic, increased secretions, pulmonary edema, ataxia, convulsions
218. ___ Initial symptoms are respiratory, respiratory alkalosis, absorption may occur from mouth, GI tract or skin, peak action occurs about 4 hours after toxic dose

Ref. 11 - pp. 1675-1678

A. Pneumococcus
B. Staphylococcus
C. Streptococcus
D. Neisseria
E. Escherichia

219. ___ Gram-positive, often in chains, produces hemolysis when cultured on sheep blood agar
220. ___ Gram-negative, intracellular, grows well on chocolate agar plates
221. ___ Gram-negative, nonsporing, lactose fermenting
222. ___ Gram-positive, "lancet" shaped, often grows in pairs
223. ___ Gram-positive, grapelike clusters, golden yellow pigmentation produced on solid agar media

Ref. 1 - pp. 766, 772, 778,
784, 792

Match item with liver function tests in differentiation of hepatogenous and obstructive jaundice:

A. Thymol turbidity
B. Transaminase
C. Cephalin flocculation
D. Alkaline phosphatase
E. Reversal of A-G ratio

224. ___ Positive in both but in varying degree
225. ___ Positive in both and not discriminatory
226. ___ Positive in hepatogenous; negative in obstructive
227. ___ Discriminatory but a late development
228. ___ More sensitive but quite non-specific

Ref. 6 - p. 1179

Match the following:

A. Ulcerative colitis
B. Crohn's disease
C. Ischemic colitis
D. Lymphogranuloma venereum

229. ___ "Thumb-printing"
230. ___ "Cobblestone" appearance

231. ___ Pseudopolyps
232. ___ Sclerosing cholangitis
233. ___ Rectal strictures which may become malignant
Ref. 4 - pp. 960, 973-976

A. Friedreich's ataxia
B. Familial progressive spastic paraplegia
C. Dystonia musculorum deformans
D. Werdnig-Hoffman disease
E. Hungtington's chorea

234. ___ Hereditary degenerative disease, destruction of Betz cells and pyramidal tract degeneration, males affected more than females, symptoms in early childhood
235. ___ Torsion of limbs or trunk, more common in European Jews, autosomal dominant inheritance, loss of cells in basal ganglion
236. ___ Progressive hypotonia and wasting of skeletal muscle in infancy and childhood, degeneration of motor neurons, cause unknown
237. ___ Progressive choreic movements, dementia and death, atrophy of frontal lobes
238. ___ Ataxia, loss of reflexes, pes cavus, kyphoscoliosis, cardiac abnormality, nystagmus and optic atrophy
Ref. 11 - pp. 1436, 1439, 1458

A. Neoplastic meningitis
B. Cerebellopontine angle tumor
C. Tumor in the superior temporal gyrus
D. Frontal lobe tumor
E. Optic nerve glioma

239. ___ Progressive nerve deafness and tinnitus
240. ___ Anomic aphasia
241. ___ Often associated with neurofibromatosis
242. ___ Glucose less than 45, negative cultures and few signs of meningeal irritability
243. ___ Early decline in intellectual function
Ref. 2 - p. 739

A. Primary lateral sclerosis
B. Benign fasciculations
C. Amyotrophic lateral sclerosis
D. Multiple sclerosis
E. Disease found in the Mariana Islands

244. ___ Upper and lower motor neuron dysfunction, sometimes with parkinsonism
245. ___ Often seen in young adults with no EMG evidence of denervation

246. ___ Progressive spastic paraparesis with later development of internuclear ophthalmoplegia in a young adult
247. ___ Weakness and wasting of muscles, with prominent fasciculations
248. ___ Progressive spastic paraparesis in a fifty-five year old female   Ref. 2 - pp. 759-761

Match the following tumors of the pancreas:

A. Insulinoma
B. Carcinoma
C. Gastrin-secreting

249. ___ Zollinger-Ellison syndrome
250. ___ Whipple's triad
251. ___ Only cure is Whipple procedure (pancreaticoduodenectomy)
252. ___ May treat by subtotal pancreatectomy
253. ___ Only treatment is total gastrectomy
                                        Ref. 4 - pp. 1116-1117

A. Amyloidosis
B. Multiple myeloma
C. Sickle cell anemia
D. Gout
E. Hypercalcemia

254. ___ Loss of concentrating ability and papillary necrosis
255. ___ Prominent renal tubular dysfunction
256. ___ Nephrotic syndrome
257. ___ Nephrocalcinosis
258. ___ Urate calculi and pyelonephritis
                                        Ref. 1 - pp. 1419-1421

A. Lymphogranuloma venereum
B. Granuloma inguinale
C. Both
D. Neither

259. ___ Donovan body
260. ___ Venereal disease
261. ___ Frei test
262. ___ Treatment with sulfonamides
263. ___ Treatment with streptomycin   Ref. 1 - pp. 982,834

A. Subcapital femoral fracture
B. Intertrochanteric fracture
C. Both
D. Neither

264. ___ Smith-Petersen nail is used
265. ___ Other internal fixation is used
266. ___ Nonunion is common
267. ___ Residual disability is common
268. ___ Traction reduction may be used   Ref. 6 - p. 1820

A. Testicular feminizing syndrome
B. True hermaphroditism
C. Both
D. Neither

269. ___ Sex-chromatin pattern is positive
270. ___ Disorder inherited and gene transmitted by female carrier
271. ___ Ovarian tissue present
272. ___ Ambiguity of external genitalia
273. ___ Good response to androgen replacement

Ref. 11 - pp. 1362-1364

A. Tetralogy of Fallot
B. Eisenmenger syndrome
C. Both
D. Neither

274. ___ Ventricular septal defect, atrial septal defect or patent ductus arteriosus
275. ___ Cyanosis (may not be present at birth)
276. ___ Dyspnea and squatting
277. ___ Diastolic murmur loud and harsh, no systolic component
278. ___ "Coeur en sabot" on x-ray   Ref. 11 - pp. 1022-1023,
1030-1031

A. Gastric ulcer
B. Duodenal ulcer
C. Both
D. Neither

279. ___ Tendency to become carcinomatous
280. ___ Treated by control of acid factor
281. ___ Tendency to bleed, perforate or obstruct
282. ___ No rationale for vagotomy
283. ___ Ulcer bed not always excised at operation

Ref. 6 - p. 1055

A. Transurethral prostatectomy
B. Open prostatectomy
C. Both
D. Neither

284. ___ Four times higher mortality rate
285. ___ Lower incidence of impotence
286. ___ Suitable palliative procedure for cancer
287. ___ Lower incidence of incontinence
288. ___ Postoperative catheter drainage not needed

Ref. 6 - p. 1577

A. Angina pectoris
B. Myocardial infarction
C. Both
D. Neither

289. ___ The electrocardiogram may be abnormal
290. ___ Marked elevation of the SGOT, LDH and CPK occur following an attack
291. ___ Occur(s) with increased frequency in Tangier disease
292. ___ Sublingual nitroglycerine is often effective in producing relief
293. ___ Dressler's syndrome may occur following an attack
                                    Ref. 1 - pp. 1200, 1198, 640
                                                        1209

A. Primary pulmonary hypertension with hyperventilation
B. Alveolar hypoventilation
C. Both
D. Neither

294. ___ Hypoxemia
295. ___ Hypercapnia
296. ___ Hypocapnia
297. ___ Low arterial bicarbonate
298. ___ Cor pulmonale   Ref. 1 - pp. 1298, 1332

A. Aortic coarctation
B. Mitral stenosis
C. Both
D. Neither

299. ___ Left ventricular hypertrophy
300. ___ Cyanosis
301. ___ Notched ribs on X-ray
302. ___ Calcification of area involved
303. ___ Rarely congenital   Ref. 6 - pp. 696, 762

A. Granulosa plus sertoli-leydig cell
B. Ectoderm, mesoderm and endoderm
C. Dysgerminoma plus sertoli-leydig cells and/or granulosa cells
D. Sertoli-leydig cells only
E. Signet ring cells

304. ___ Gonadoblastoma
305. ___ Gynandroblastoma
306. ___ Arrhenoblastoma
307. ___ Krukenberg
308. ___ Teratoma   Ref. 8 - pp. 513, 533,
                                                 528, 493,
                                                 502

After each of the following case histories there is a series of
multiple choice questions based on the history. Select the one
most appropriate answer:

CASE (Questions 309-312): A 17-year-old primigravida at term enters
in labor with 2 cm cervical dilatation and the vertex at -3 station.
Pelvimetry is done and the X-rays show a flat sacrum and a biischial
spinous diameter of 7 cm.

309. This would constitute:
 A. Inlet contracture
 B. Outlet contracture
 C. Midpelvic contracture
 D. A juxta minor pelvis
 E. None of the above
 Ref. 7 - p. 907

310. Forceps operations with this type of pelvis are difficult because:
 A. The head commonly presents as a posterior
 B. The head presents with anterior asynclitism
 C. Forceps pull destroys flexion of the head
 D. Forceps pull destroys extension of the head
 E. None of the above
 Ref. 7 - pp. 907-908

311. If dystocia occurs the best method of delivery would probably
 be:
 A. High forceps delivery
 B. Stimulation by pitocin
 C. C-section
 D. Version and extraction
 E. None of the above
 Ref. 7 - p. 907

312. The mother's gonadal dose in the pelvimetry done would be:
 A. 2-4 r
 B. 8-10 r
 C. 10-12 r
 D. 14-16 r
 E. 16-18 r
 Ref. 7 - p. 317

CASE (Questions 313-316): A 35-year-old man has been complaining
of tinnitus and vertigo for three years. He also noted that his hearing
has become progressively worse on the right side. On examination
he was found to have an unsteady gait and impairment of hearing on
the right side. Several 2 cm x 2 cm firm movable nontender nodules
were found in the upper part of his back. A biopsy of the nodule con-
firmed his physician's clinical diagnosis.

313. The most probable cause of his complaints is:
 A. Menière's disease
 B. Otitis media
 C. Acoustic neurofibroma
 D. Vestibular neuronitis
 E. Goodpasture's syndrome

314. An X-ray of the skull taken to aid in the diagnosis probably will
 reveal:
 A. No abnormality
 B. Erosion of the internal auditory meatus
 C. Mastoiditis
 D. Calcification of the basal ganglia
 E. Enlarged sella turcica

315. Biopsy of the skin nodule probably revealed:
 A. Lipoma
 B. Melanoma
 C. Osteoma
 D. Necrotic tissue with foreign body giant cells
 E. Neurofibroma

316. Amelioration of his illness is best achieved by:
 A. Tetracycline
 B. Craniotomy
 C. Idoxuridine
 D. Dramamine
 E. Chloramphenicol ear drops
 Ref. 2 - p. 767

CASE (Questions 317-320): A 40-year-old female was seen because of varicose veins.

317. This condition may be caused most commonly by:
 A. High systemic arterial pressure
 B. Prolonged ingestion of aspirin
 C. Defective valves in veins
 D. Herniation of the intervertebral disc
 E. None of the above

318. The manifestations of this disorder may include:
 A. Edema of the legs
 B. Increased pigmentation of the legs
 C. Ulcers of the legs
 D. Stasis dermatitis
 E. All of the above

319. Each of the following conditions may aggravate the ailment, except:
 A. Pregnancy
 B. Thrombophlebitis
 C. Excessive weight loss
 D. Ascites
 E. Abdominal tumor

320. Management of this patient may include each of the following, except:
 A. Injection of sclerosing substances
 B. Tight panty girdle
 C. Ligation and stripping of the veins
 D. Elastic stockings
 E. Elevation of the feet during sleep
 Ref. 2 - p. 1083

CASE (Questions 321-324): As an 18-year-old girl was crossing the street, a car slowing for the red traffic light struck her from the left side, the bumper hitting her at the knee. She had immediate inability to extend and flex the knee which was in a marked valgus position.

321. The most probable diagnosis is fracture of:
 A. Lateral tibial condyle
 B. Both tibial condyles
 C. Medial tibial condyle
 D. Patella
 E. Femoral condyles

322. Proper maneuver in reduction and fixation is:
    A. Medial pressure to a slightly varus position
    B. Compress fragments medially with a C-clamp
    C. Apply cast from toes to groin
    D. Check position of fragments by post-cast X-ray
    E. All of the above

323. Post-reduction X-ray shows the fragment to be depressed and not maneuverable. Treatment is any, except:
    A. Elevate fragment and hold by capsular sutures
    B. Elevate fragment and hold by screws
    C. Excise the fragment
    D. Lever the plateau up and fill defect with bone chips

324. Open operation may show any, except which additional injury?
    A. Collateral ligament   D. Semilunar cartilage
    B. Fibular head   E. Cruciate ligament
    C. Joint cartilage   Ref. 4 - p. 1358

CASE (Questions 325-328): A 62-year-old man had been having increasing difficulty with defecation because of pain, bleeding and narrowed anal orifice. There was an ulcerated area just below the pectinate line on the left.

325. You suspect malignancy and order which test?
    A. Barium enema   D. Liver scintogram
    B. Proctosigmoidoscopy   E. Inguinal node biopsy
    C. Biopsy at ulcer margin

326. Biopsy reveals squamous cell cancer of the anus so you realize that all are true, except:
    A. Extension upward is not likely
    B. Liver metastases will be unusual
    C. Local extension is frequent
    D. Metastases will be to regional inguinal nodes
    E. Radium application will control the local lesion

327. The approved therapy in this case is:
    A. Radium pack application
    B. Local excision and proctoplasty
    C. Combined abdomino-perineal excision
    D. Combined abdomino-perineal excision with inguinal node dissection
    E. Diverting colostomy and later local cauterization

328. The conventional combined abdomino-perineal resection here is varied to:
    A. Remove more perianal skin
    B. Retain the sphincter
    C. Remove ischiorectal fat and nodes
    D. Do en-bloc dissection with the groin
    E. Leave the wound open for X-ray therapy
                                    Ref. 6 - pp. 1159-1160

CASE (Questions 329-332): A 20-year-old man complained of difficulty in breathing for the past six months. He did not have any history of cough or expectoration.. There was no history of any cardiac illness in the past. He is a nonsmoker. He used to participate actively in sports until 4 years ago when he started having low back pain especially in the mornings. These pains were worse on coughing or straining. He consulted a physician who told the patient that he had sacroiliitis on X-ray. For approximately 3 months he noticed that he was having dyspnea on exertion and difficulty in bending forwards or backwards. At the same time he developed photophobia and pain in both eyes. The physician who saw him at this time gave him some eye drops.

On examination the patient was not in any acute distress. There was no cyanosis, jaundice or paleness of the mucosa. His pupils were unequal in size, but reacted normally to light and accommodation. Blood pressure 160/60 mm Hg. Pulse 90/min and regular. Temperature normal. Examination of the chest revealed restrictive mobility but was otherwise normal. Cardiac examination revealed a short diastolic murmur. The patient experienced difficulty in bending forwards or backwards. Examination of the spine revealed some localized tenderness at the right sacroiliac area. Laboratory data were all normal except for elevated sedimentation rate. Urinalysis, normal. EKG revealed left ventricular hypertrophy.

329. The probable diagnosis of this young man's illness is:
   A. Rheumatoid arthritis   D. Reiter's syndrome
   B. Paget's disease   E. Ankylosing spondylitis
   C. Fluorosis

330. The diastolic murmur heard in the heart is probably due to:
   A. Aortic regurgitation   D. Pulmonary regurgitation
   B. Mitral stenosis   E. Austin Flint murmur
   C. Tricuspid stenosis

331. X-ray of the spine most probably will show:
   A. Markedly decreased density of all the vertebral bodies with "fish mouth appearance"
   B. Osteolytic and osteoblastic areas of the vertebral bodies
   C. "Bamboo spine" and destruction of sacroiliac joints
   D. Cervical spondylosis
   E. Subluxation of the lumbar vertebrae

332. The low back pain occurring in this disorder often responds well to:
   A. Gold salts   D. Phenylbutazone
   B. Calcitonin   E. Penicillin
   C. Tetracycline   Ref. 2 - p. 150

CASE (Questions 333-336): A 12-year-old girl was found on routine examination to have a systolic murmur at the 2nd left intercostal space. There was wide splitting of the second heart sound which did not change during respiration. The pulmonic component was louder than the aortic component. EKG revealed right ventricular hypertrophy and right bundle branch block.

333. The most probable diagnosis is:
    A. Pulmonary stenosis
    B. Interatrial septal defect
    C. Interventricular septal defect
    D. Hypertrophic aortic stenosis
    E. Mitral regurgitation

334. The right bundle branch block in this patient is due to:
    A. Right atrial hypertrophy
    B. Frequent pulmonary emboli
    C. Associated pulmonary stenosis
    D. Associated tricuspid incompetence
    E. None of the above

335. X-ray of the chest will probably reveal:
    A. Prominent pulmonary arteries
    B. Oligemic lung fields
    C. Multiple shadows due to pulmonary emboli
    D. Dilated aorta
    E. Giant left atrium

336. Early in its course this disorder is usually an example of:
    A. Right-to-left shunt
    B. Left-to-right shunt
    C. Bidirectional shunt
    D. No intracardiac shunt
    E. A systolic left-to-right and a diastolic right-to-left shunt
                                        Ref. 2 - p. 944

CASE (Questions 337-340): A 4-year-old child is seen by a pediatrician with a chief complaint of fever, loss of appetite, lack of energy and pallor. The youngster had been in good health. On examination petechiae are discovered. Moderate painless adenopathy is detected. Mild hepatomegaly and moderate splenic enlargement are palpated. The youngster is hospitalized and that evening complains of bone pain.

337. The most likely diagnosis is:
    A. Rheumatoid arthritis   D. Infectious mononucleosis
    B. Rheumatic fever   E. Influenza
    C. Acute leukemia

338. The most useful examination would be:
   A. Skull X-rays
   B. Lumbar puncture
   C. Blood culture
   D. Urine analysis
   E. Bone marrow

339. If a diagnosis of acute leukemia were established, the prognosis for an 18 month survival is approximately ___ per cent.
   A. 10
   B. 15
   C. 25
   D. 35
   E. 50

340. 70 per cent of deaths are due to:
   A. Infection
   B. Hemorrhage
   C. Convulsions
   D. Cardiac tamponade
   E. Respiratory arrest
   Ref. 10 - pp. 1208-1213

CASE (Questions 341-344): A 32-year-old mother of three had noticed a dark discoloration under her right thumbnail for the past six months. The nail finally came off and was replaced by a draining ulcerated area with enlarged nodes appearing in the axilla.

341. The probable diagnosis is:
   A. Chronic felon
   B. Melanoma
   C. Phalangeal osteomyelitis
   D. Subungual hematoma
   E. Glomus tumor

342. Adequate diagnosis is established by:
   A. Search of blood smears for melanocytes
   B. Typical X-ray appearance of the thumb
   C. Response to chemotherapy
   D. Biopsy of the lesion and an enlarged axillary node
   E. Trial therapy with X-ray

343. The only chance for cure in this case, in the absence of evident metastasis beyond the axilla is:
   A. Amputation of the thumb and axillary dissection
   B. Heavy X-ray therapy to lesion, arm and axilla
   C. Forequarter amputation and radical axillary dissection
   D. Laser destruction of lesion followed by chemotherapy
   E. Cure is out of the question; only palliation is possible

344. Within a year after treatment, there are pulmonary and hepatic metastases, requiring which palliative method?
   A. X-ray therapy
   B. Adrenalectomy
   C. No treatment is worthwhile
   D. Chemotherapy
   E. Only symptomatic care
   Ref. 6 - p. 523

CASE (Questions 345-348): On physical examination of a 19-year-old draftee, elevated blood pressure was discovered, with visible neck pulsations and a murmur over most of the left hemithorax.

345. What other physical finding should be expected?
    A. Decreased or absent lower extremity pulses
    B. Palpable and visible pulsations in the shoulder muscles
    C. Lower blood pressure in the legs
    D. Heavy pulsation in retinal arteries
    E. All of the above

346. Chest X-ray will show:
    A. Reverse "3" sign at lower right mediastinal border
    B. Dilatation of the right heart
    C. Notching of lower borders of ribs
    D. Site of aortic obstruction
    E. Pulmonary congestion

347. Your diagnosis is:
    A. Aortic coarctation   D. Patent ductus arteriosus
    B. Aortic stenosis   E. Over-riding of the aorta
    C. Vascular ring

348. Aortography:
    A. Will demonstrate any other congenital defects
    B. Is not needed in most cases of coaractation
    C. Is too risky to use in coarctation
    D. Is more valuable than cardiac catheterization if other lesions
       are suspected
    E. Is contraindicated if there is calcification
                                    Ref. 6 - pp. 696-697

CASE (Questions 349-352): A 60-year-old male complains of severe
mid-epigastric pain of several years duration. A peptic ulcer had
been diagnosed previously, but the patient's symptoms were not im-
proved by a good medical regimen. Furthermore, after partial
gastrectomy,recurrent ulceration developed. More recently the
patient has complained of profuse watery diarrhea.

349. The fundamental disorder in this patient is most likely due to:
    A. Thyroid adenoma
    B. Non-beta islet cell adenoma of the pancreas
    C. Giant hypertrophy of the gastric mucosa
    D. Carcinoid tumor of the intestine
    E. Excessive smoking

350. The concentration of which of the following is most likely to
    be increased in serum?
    A. Hydrochloric acid   D. Cortisone
    B. Thyroid hormone   E. Amylase
    C. Gastrin

351. The basal secretion of hydrochloric acid is most likely to be:
    A. Normal
    B. Slightly decreased
    C. Greatly increased
    D. Slightly increased
    E. Greatly decreased but sti-
       mulated 2-fold by histamine

352. The treatment of choice in this patient probably would be:
    A. Intensive psychotherapy
    B. Neck dissection
    C. Vagotomy
    D. Gastroenterostomy
    E. Total gastrectomy
       Ref. 2 - p. 1209

CASE (Questions 353-356): A 48-year-old woman had a Wertheim hysterectomy 8 months ago. She now has a soft cystic 3-4 cm mass near the right lateral pelvic wall.

353. The most likely diagnosis is:
    A. Recurrent carcinoma
    B. Diverticulum of the bladder
    C. Pelvic lymphocyst
    D. Sacculation of the ureter
    E. Pelvic abscess

354. The etiology of this lesion post pelvic radical surgery is:
    A. Pre-operative radiation
    B. Excess accumulation of blood postoperatively
    C. Postoperative infection
    D. All of the above
    E. None of the above

355. The most serious threat posed by this lesion is:
    A. Infection
    B. Wound dehiscence
    C. Ureteral obstruction
    D. Bowel obstruction
    E. Hemorrhage

356. The diagnosis of this lesion may be best accomplished with:
    A. Flat plate of abdomen
    B. Aspiration
    C. Exclusion diagnosis
    D. Pelvic lymphangioadeno-
       graphy
    E. None of the above
       Ref. 9 - p. 597

For each of the questions or incomplete statements below, one or more of the answers or completions given is correct. Answer according to the following key:

A. If only 1, 2 and 3 are correct
B. If only 1 and 3 are correct
C. If only 2 and 4 are correct
D. If only 4 is correct
E. If all are correct

357. Lowered blood calcium levels in cases of acute pancreatitis point to:
    1. Retroperitoneal edema
    2. Diaphragmatic irritation
    3. Pancreatic rupture
    4. Severe form of the disease   Ref. 6 - p. 1262

358. In incarcerated inguinal hernia, which of the following suggests the presence of non-viable bowel?
    1. Signs of peritoneal irritation
    2. Hypoactive or absent bowel sounds
    3. Scrotal inflammation
    4. Tender sac and abdominal tenderness
                                Ref. 6 - pp. 1346-1350

359. Preferred treatment of rectal and colonic polyps is by:
    1. Segmental resection if stalk shows cancer
    2. Segmental resection if polyp is sessile
    3. Polypectomy if stalk is clear on frozen section
    4. Fulguration if one cm or less in diameter
                                Ref. 6 - p. 1128

360. Defects in operative cholangiograms, caused by air bubbles, may be recognized by:
    1. Lack of deformation of the duct contour
    2. Uniform radiolucency without lamination
    3. Tendency to be perfectly spherical
    4. Multiple shadows in all cases   Ref. 6 - p. 1230

ANSWER KEY

1. E	51. C	101. E	151. C	201. B
2. C	52. B	102. C	152. B	202. E
3. B	53. A	103. C	153. A	203. C
4. C	54. D	104. D	154. C	204. B
5. C	55. B	105. E	155. D	205. A
6. D	56. E	106. B	156. B	206. C
7. A	57. B	107. E	157. B	207. A
8. D	58. E	108. B	158. C	208. A
9. D	59. D	109. D	159. B	209. A
10. C	60. E	110. E	160. E	210. A
11. E	61. B	111. D	161. A	211. B
12. C	62. D	112. E	162. B	212. D
13. D	63. D	113. B	163. B	213. B
14. C	64. C	114. B	164. B	214. E
15. C	65. E	115. A	165. C	215. A
16. A	66. B	116. C	166. C	216. B
17. D	67. D	117. C	167. D	217. C
18. B	68. E	118. A	168. D	218. D
19. B	69. A	119. B	169. D	219. C
20. B	70. D	120. A	170. B	220. D
21. E	71. C	121. E	171. C	221. E
22. C	72. D	122. C	172. D	222. A
23. E	73. B	123. E	173. A	223. B
24. D	74. B	124. E	174. A	224. C
25. C	75. D	125. C	175. C	225. D
26. A	76. E	126. A	176. B	226. A
27. B	77. B	127. B	177. C	227. E
28. C	78. E	128. E	178. D	228. B
29. C	79. A	129. A	179. E	229. C
30. A	80. C	130. C	180. B	230. B
31. B	81. C	131. E	181. C	231. A
32. E	82. C	132. E	182. C	232. A
33. A	83. C	133. D	183. A	233. D
34. D	84. B	134. E	184. B	234. B
35. E	85. D	135. D	185. C	235. C
36. C	86. C	136. C	186. D	236. D
37. C	87. D	137. D	187. E	237. E
38. E	88. C	138. E	188. C	238. A
39. C	89. D	139. D	189. B	239. B
40. E	90. D	140. B	190. C	240. C
41. D	91. C	141. E	191. E	241. E
42. C	92. A	142. A	192. A	242. A
43. A	93. A	143. D	193. D	243. D
44. D	94. A	144. E	194. E	244. E
45. E	95. A	145. D	195. D	245. B
46. D	96. E	146. A	196. C	246. D
47. B	97. B	147. B	197. A	247. C
48. E	98. E	148. C	198. B	248. A
49. D	99. D	149. B	199. D	249. C
50. D	100. E	150. C	200. A	250. A

ANSWER KEY

251. B	301. A	351. C
252. A	302. C	352. E
253. C	303. B	353. C
254. C	304. C	354. D
255. B	305. A	355. C
256. A	306. D	356. D
257. E	307. E	357. D
258. D	308. B	358. E
259. B	309. C	359. E
260. C	310. C	360. A
261. A	311. C	
262. A	312. A	
263. B	313. C	
264. D	314. B	
265. B	315. E	
266. A	316. B	
267. C	317. C	
268. C	318. E	
269. B	319. C	
270. A	320. B	
271. B	321. A	
272. B	322. E	
273. D	323. C	
274. B	324. B	
275. C	325. C	
276. C	326. E	
277. D	327. D	
278. A	328. A	
279. D	329. E	
280. B	330. A	
281. C	331. C	
282. A	332. D	
283. B	333. B	
284. B	334. E	
285. A	335. A	
286. C	336. A	
287. A	337. C	
288. D	338. E	
289. C	339. E	
290. B	340. A	
291. D	341. B	
292. A	342. D	
293. B	343. C	
294. C	344. D	
295. B	345. E	
296. A	346. C	
297. A	347. A	
298. C	348. B	
299. A	349. B	
300. D	350. C	

FOURTH EXAMINATION

For each of the following multiple choice questions, select the one most appropriate answer:

1. Metabolic alkalosis associated with prolonged vomiting or nasogastric suction is due primarily to loss of:
   A. Sodium
   B. Potassium
   C. Chloride
   D. Hydrogen ion
   E. Bicarbonate
   Ref. 4 - p. 105

2. After spinal cord injury, the most important test indicating need for decompressive laminectomy is:
   A. Myelography
   B. Plain X-ray of spine
   C. Queckenstedt test
   D. Pneumomyelography
   E. Ultrasound
   Ref. 6 - p. 1642

3. In causalgia, the two nerves most commonly affected are:
   A. Median and sciatic
   B. Ulnar and peroneal
   C. Radial and spinal accessory
   D. Vagus and parasympathetic
   E. Iliohypogastric and sural
   Ref. 6 - p. 1977

4. The reason for a three weeks waiting period before repair of peripheral nerve severance is:
   A. The wound will be clean and healed
   B. Extent of nerve injury can be identified more precisely
   C. Schwann cell proliferation is optimal for reestablishing continuity of the neurolemmal tubules
   D. Sutures hold better in the thickened epineurium
   E. All of the above
   Ref. 4 - p. 1307

5. Which statement is false as regards response to trauma?
   A. 17-hydroxycorticoid excretion is increased after stress
   B. Increase in 17-hydroxycorticoids corresponds to decrease in eosinophiles
   C. Increased steroid excretion is accompanied by decreased nitrogen excretion
   D. All adrenocorticoid excretion is increased after stress
   E. After four days, steroid excretion and nitrogen loss do not correlate
   Ref. 4 - p. 40

6. Which statement is true regarding exploration for hyperparathyroidism?
   A. The clear-cell hyperplasia is smooth, vascular and reddish-brown
   B. The adenoma is dark chocolate colored and irregular
   C. A missing lower pole gland will be found in the anterior mediastinum
   D. A missing upper pole gland will be found antero-superiorly
   E. In hyperplasia, removal of two glands is sufficient
   Ref. 6 - p. 1458

7. In women with heart disease, which stage of labor is most poorly tolerated?
    A. First
    B. Second
    C. Third
    D. Fourth
    E. All stages
    Ref. 9 - p. 262

8. Premature infants are especially liable in the neonatal period to:
    A. Respiratory problems
    B. Cerebral hemorrhage
    C. Anemia
    D. Kernicterus
    E. All of the above
    Ref. 9 - pp. 359-360

9. Which is important in the diagnosis of ruptured membranes prior to labor:
    A. Careful history
    B. Nitrazine test
    C. Amniotic fluid crystallization test
    D. Nile blue stain
    E. All of the above
    Ref. 9 - p. 363

10. Drugs definitely associated with fetal anomalies:
    A. Aspirin
    B. Prednisone
    C. Valium
    D. Antifolic acid compounds
    E. Erythromycin
    Ref. 7 - p. 1067

11. Weinberg's sign is a radiologic finding in:
    A. Uterine anomalies
    B. Abdominal pregnancy
    C. Dermoid cysts
    D. Rh isoimmunization
    E. None of the above
    Ref. 9 - p. 233

12. The rate of amniotic fluid turnover is:
    A. 100 cc/hour
    B. 200 cc/hour
    C. 300 cc/hour
    D. 400 cc/hour
    E. 500 cc/hour
    Ref. 7 - p. 227

13. The arias-stella phenomenon is seen in:
    A. Endometrial carcinoma
    B. Ovarian serous cystadenoma
    C. Cervical endometriosis
    D. Ectopic pregnancy
    E. Endometriosis
    Ref. 8 - pp. 572-576

14. The incubation period for rabies may be as long as:
    A. One week
    B. One month
    C. Three months
    D. Six months
    E. One year
    Ref. 2 - p. 702

15. Neuropathic joint disease may develop in:
    A. Tabes dorsalis
    B. Diabetes
    C. Syringomyelia
    D. All of the above
    E. None of the above
    Ref. 1 - p. 2012

16. Which one of the following diseases is not treated with amphotericin B?
    A. Histoplasmosis
    B. Nocardiosis
    C. Coccidioidomycosis
    D. Mucormycosis
    E. Cryptococcosis
    Ref. 1 - p. 906

17. Disease caused by the fusospirochetal infections may include:
    A. Granuloma inguinale   D. Vincent's angina
    B. Lymphogranuloma venereum   E. All of the above
    C. Chancroid   Ref. 1 - p. 840

18. Findings in a patient with pertussis may include:
    A. Epistaxis   D. Convulsions
    B. Ulcers of the tongue   E. All of the above
    C. Lymphocytosis   Ref. 1 - p. 816

19. Which one of the following statements is not true of respiratory
    infection due to H. influenzae?
    A. Pneumonia due to this organism is common in children
    B. Bronchitis can be a manifestation of the infection
    C. Bronchiolitis can be a manifestation of the infection
    D. The organisms are uniformly resistant to ampicillin
    E. The organisms are frequently isolated from the respiratory
       tracts of individuals with established chronic bronchitis
                                          Ref. 1 - p. 814

20. Which one of the following is characteristic of streptococcal
    pneumonia?
    A. Lack of fever   D. Absence of organisms in
    B. Interstitial pneumonia   the sputum
    C. Leukopenia   E. Absence of cough
                                 Ref. 1 - p. 782

21. Parathormone and thyrocalcitonin have an effect on:
    A. Integrity of bone
    B. Sensitivity of nerves
    C. Excretory function of the kidneys
    D. Excretory function of the large bowel
    E. All of the above   Ref. 6 - p. 1464

22. Diffuse toxic goiter and nodular toxic goiter are alike in:
    A. Tendency to cardiac decompensation
    B. Age incidence
    C. Incidence of exophthalmos
    D. Symptoms
    E. Occurrence of thyroid crisis   Ref. 6 - p. 1439

23. Thyroid hyperplasia is controlled by use of:
    A. Pituitary extract   D. Sympatheticomimetic drugs
    B. Desiccated thyroid   E. Radioisotopes
    C. Catecholamines   Ref. 6 - p. 1447

24. All of the following are true about tetralogy of Fallot patients
    except:
    A. They are cyanotic at birth   D. They have decreased lung
    B. They often squat   vascularity on X-ray
    C. They have clubbing of fingers E. 25% have right aortic arch
                                        Ref. 4 - p. 1991

25. The operation for definitive correction of transposition of the great vessels is:
    A. Blalock-Taussig procedure
    B. Potts procedure
    C. Waterston procedure
    D. Mustard procedure
    E. Rashkind procedure
    Ref. 4 - p. 2009

26. Which of the following rule out radical mastectomy for breast cancer?
    A. Satellite nodules over breast skin
    B. Parasternal tumor nodules
    C. Proven supraclavicular metastasis
    D. Edema of the arm
    E. All of the above
    Ref. 6 - p. 541

27. Glomus tumor:
    A. Is most frequent along the anterior shin
    B. Is made up of lymph vessels and adipose tissue
    C. Is painful because it contains myelinated nerve fibers
    D. Occurs as red to purple nodules under digital nails
    E. Is treated by irradiation
    Ref. 6 - p. 518

28. Which one of the following is usually not a feature of chronic constrictive pericarditis?
    A. Dyspnea on exertion
    B. Frequent attacks of acute pulmonary edema
    C. Distended neck veins
    D. Distant heart sounds
    E. Low voltage QRS complexes on EKG
    Ref. 1 - p. 1216

29. A bloody pericardial effusion may be due to:
    A. Tuberculous pericarditis
    B. Tumor involving the pericardium
    C. Uremic pericarditis
    D. All of the above
    E. None of the above
    Ref. 1 - p. 1212

30. The valvular lesion most often resulting from myocardial infarction is:
    A. Aortic stenosis
    B. Aortic insufficiency
    C. Mitral regurgitation
    D. Mitral stenosis
    E. Pulmonary stenosis
    Ref. 1 - p. 1200

31. In the Keith-Wagener-Barker classification of hypertensive and arteriosclerotic retinopathy, the presence of exudates and hemorrhages without papilledema is classified as ____ retinopathy:
    A. Normal
    B. Grade I
    C. Grade II
    D. Grade III
    E. Grade IV
    Ref. 1 - p. 190

32. Which one of the following disorders is usually characterized by systolic hypertension only?
    A. Chronic pyelonephritis
    B. Patent ductus arteriosus
    C. Polycystic renal disease
    D. Renovascular hypertension
    E. Diabetic nephropathy
    Ref. 1 - p. 1160

33. Causes of secondary polycythemia may include:
    A. Renal carcinoma
    B. Cerebellar hemangioblastoma
    C. Pheochromocytoma
    D. All of the above
    E. None of the above
    Ref. 1 - p. 175 -176

34. The half-life of transfused platelets is approximately:
    A. 4-5 days
    B. 36-48 hours
    C. 8-10 hours
    D. 7-8 days
    E. None of the above
    Ref. 1 - p. 1638

35. In severe burns, respiratory distress may be due to:
    A. Edema from burns of upper airway
    B. Pulmonary edema from burn or fluid overload
    C. Pneumonia secondary to septicemia
    D. Inhibition of respiratory excursion by tight eschar
    E. Any of the above
    Ref. 6 - p. 258

36. In figuring colloid requirement for the first 24 hours after serious thermal injury, which of the following is correct?
    A. 1 ml/Kg body wt/% body surface burn
    B. 0.5 ml/Kg body wt/% body surface burn
    C. 1.5 ml/Kg body wt/% body surface burn
    D. Double the amount if low molecular dextran is used
    E. Increase the amount by 1/3 in hot weather
    Ref. 6 - p. 261

37. Damage to the tail of the pancreas should be treated by:
    A. Drainage alone
    B. Primary suture and drainage
    C. Primary suture alone
    D. Resection of the tail and drainage
    E. Resection of the tail, ligation of the main pancreatic duct, and drainage
    Ref. 4 - p. 382

38. Causes of death in untreated coarctation of the aorta include all of the following, except:
    A. Bacterial endocarditis or aortitis
    B. Rupture of the aorta
    C. Myocardial infarction
    D. Congestive heart failure
    E. Cerebrovascular accident
    Ref. 4 - p. 1939

39. The most common type of malignant tumor of the renal pelvis and ureter is:
    A. Papillary carcinoma
    B. Transitional cell papilloma
    C. Squamous cell cancer
    D. Adenocarcinoma
    E. Sarcoma
    Ref. 6 - p. 1571

40. If the epididymis is hard, irregular, enlarged and fixed but not particularly tender, the diagnosis probably is:
    A. Syphilis
    B. Gonorrhea
    C. Neoplasm
    D. Tuberculosis
    E. Actinomycosis
    Ref. 4 - p. 1568

41. A frequent complication of acute or chronic prostatitis is:
    A. Epididymitis
    B. Orchitis
    C. Cystocele
    D. Sterility
    E. Seminal vesiculitis
    Ref. 4 - p. 1567

42. Sclerodermatous involvement of the heart may lead to:
    A. Cardiomyopathy
    B. Pericarditis
    C. Heart block
    D. All of the above
    E. None of the above
    Ref. 1 - p. 2010

43. The features of thalassemia major may include:
    A. Enlarged spleen
    B. Target cells in the peripheral blood smear
    C. A mongoloid appearance
    D. Reduced osmotic fragility
    E. All of the above
    Ref. 1 - p. 1622

44. The porphyrin present in normal erythrocyte hemoglobin is:
    A. Coproporphyrin I
    B. Uroporphyrin III
    C. Protoporphyrin III
    D. Uroporphyrin I
    E. Coproporphyrin III
    Ref. 1 - p. 291

45. The "direct" Coombs test is usually positive during a hemolytic episode associated with:
    A. Paroxysmal cold hemoglobinuria
    B. Paroxysmal nocturnal hemoglobinuria
    C. Hereditary spherocytosis
    D. Thalassemia
    E. None of the above
    Ref. 1 - p. 1613

46. The minimal amount of methemoglobin in the blood generally required in order to produce recognizable cyanosis is:
    A. 100 mg
    B. 250 mg
    C. 10 gm
    D. 1.5 gm
    E. None of the above
    Ref. 1 - p. 1645

47. Decreased secretion of which trophic hormone of the anterior pituitary gland is most commonly observed in cases of anorexia nervosa?
    A. ACTH
    B. Growth hormone
    C. Gonadotrophin
    D. TSH
    E. None of the above
    Ref. 2 - p. 1386

48. A drug which prevents uric acid synthesis by inhibiting the enzyme xanthine oxidase is:
    A. Colchicine
    B. Phenylbutazone
    C. Allopurinol
    D. Probenecid
    E. High doses of salicylates
    Ref. 1 - p. 616

49. Factors associated with increased risk of breast carcinoma include all of the following, except:
    A. Low parity
    B. First pregnancy after age 20
    C. Immediate relative with breast carcinoma
    D. Previous contralateral breast carcinoma
    E. Oophorectomy by age 40
    Ref. 4 - p. 581

50. Transurethral prostatic resection:
    A. Carries a high mortality in elderly men
    B. Is especially successful for median bar hypertrophy
    C. Carries a high incidence of impotence
    D. Can be combined with bladder tumor fulguration
    E. Not indicated in prostatic cancer
    Ref. 6 - p. 1577

51. The incidence of carcinoma of the thyroid in nodular goiter is:
    A. Less than 20%
    B. 25%
    C. 50%
    D. 75%
    E. 90%
    Ref. 4 - p. 632

52. Patients with esophageal hiatus hernia also often have:
    A. Pancreatitis
    B. Diverticulitis
    C. Zenker's diverticulum
    D. Duodenal ulcer
    E. Carcinoma of the colon
    Ref. 4 - p. 750

53. Which statement regarding hallux valgus is correct?
    A. The exostosis is due to chronic infection of the bursa
    B. Holding the great toe in an adducted position is curative
    C. The laterally displaced extensor tendon acts as a bow-string
    D. The inflamed bursa is due to an exostosis beneath it
    E. Produces a typical waddling gait
    Ref. 6 - p. 1868

54. Corrected position in talipes equinovarus is attained by:
    A. Forefoot abduction and pronation
    B. Eversion of the heel
    C. Dorsiflexion of the foot
    D. All of the above
    E. None of the above
    Ref. 6 - p. 1732

55. Keratoses on the hand:
    A. Should be excised
    B. Are premalignant
    C. Usually are on sun-exposed surfaces
    D. Occur predominantly in older persons
    E. All of the above   Ref. 6 - p. 517

56. Hypertrophic osteoarthropathy is characterized by:
    A. Lack of pain even in the presence of advanced changes
    B. Development only in the presence of clubbed digits
    C. Primarily proximal involvement of the long bones
    D. All of the above
    E. None of the above   Ref. 1 - p. 2011

57. Common symptoms of acute adrenal insufficiency include:
    A. Fever   D. All of the above
    B. Abdominal pain   E. None of the above
    C. Shock   Ref. 1 - p. 515

58. Advantages of evaporated milk in infant feedings:
    A. Can keep for months in unopened cans without refrigeration
    B. Casein curd in stomach softer and smaller than that of boiled
       whole milk
    C. Lactalbumin less allergenic than fresh milk
    D. All of the above
    E. None of the above   Ref. 11 - p. 172

59. All of the following are clinical disturbances due to pyridoxine
    deficiency, except:
    A. Convulsions in infants   D. Dermatitis
    B. Uveitis and cataracts   E. Anemia
    C. Peripheral neuritis   Ref. 11 - p. 194

60. All of the following are undesirable side-effects of diphenylhy-
    dantoin therapy, except:
    A. Respiratory alkalosis   D. Granulocytopenia
    B. Gingival hyperplasia   E. Megaloblastic anemia
    C. Hirsutism   Ref. 11 - p. 1743

61. All of the following are inherited as dominant traits, except:
    A. Epidermolysis bullosa simplex
    B. Multiple exostoses
    C. Hepatolenticular degeneration (Wilson's disease)
    D. Neurofibromatosis
    E. Hemorrhagic telangiectasia   Ref. 11 - p. 294

62. Major clinical findings associated with 13-trisomy syndrome:
    A. Microcephaly   D. Malformed ears
    B. Cleft lip   E. All of the above
    C. Single palmar crease   Ref. 11 - p. 305

63. Human bite infections of the hand are especially serious because:
   A. Staphylococci are present
   B. There are spirochetes present
   C. Streptococci are present
   D. Organisms are virulent and immediately invasive
   E. All of the above   Ref. 4 - p. 347

64. The incidence of esophageal carcinoma in patients who have previously suffered a lye stricture is ___ that of the normal population:
   A. 10%   D. 100 times
   B. The same as   E. 1000 times
   C. 10 times   Ref. 4 - p. 759

65. In treatment of stress ulcer, the operation of choice is:
   A. Vagotomy and pyloroplasty   D. Total gastrectomy
   B. Vagotomy and antrectomy   E. Wedge resection of the ulcer
   C. Subtotal gastrectomy   Ref. 4 - p. 843

66. In the process of bone healing:
   A. Acid phosphatase increases at fracture site after 10-14 days
   B. Calcification of hematoma is initial process in bone repair
   C. Periosteum, endosteum and fibroblasts all have osteogenic functions
   D. After 48 hours, fracture reduction is easier because muscle spasm abates
   E. The speed of new bone formation is governed by Wolff's law
                                   Ref. 4 - p. 1328

67. Which of the following is not true about squatting?
   A. Decreases peripheral vascular resistance
   B. Increases pulmonary flow
   C. Most common in tetralogy of Fallot
   D. Common in cyanotic heart disease children
   E. Associated with exertional dyspnea
                                   Ref. 6 - p. 681

68. If Crohn's disease is discovered on laparotomy for suspected appendicitis, one should:
   A. Biopsy the small bowel, alone
   B. Biopsy the small bowel and do appendectomy
   C. Do appendectomy alone
   D. Do nothing
   E. Do proximal diverting ileostomy
                                   Ref. 4 - p. 900

69. A diagnosis of mitral stenosis can be made with certainty on finding:
   A. Opening snap   D. Increased first sound
   B. Apical diastolic rumble E. All of the above
   C. Enlarged left atrium   Ref. 6 - p. 766

70. A 12 hour old infant exhibits jaundice; the most likely cause is:
    A. "Physiologic"   D. Galactosemia
    B. Erythroblastosis fetalis   E. Hepatitis
    C. Septicemia   Ref. 11 - p. 351

71. Which one of the following is a nonpreventable infection acquired
    during gestation:
    A. Syphilis   D. Toxoplasmosis
    B. Tuberculosis   E. Vaccinia
    C. Poliomyelitis   Ref. 11 - p. 399

72. Ankylosing spondylitis is usually associated with:
    A. Peripheral arthritis usually involving large joints (knees,
       ankles, hips)
    B. Heel pain is common
    C. Characteristic involvement of sacroiliac joints
    D. Deformity of peripheral joints is uncommon
    E. All of the above   Ref. 11 - pp. 531-532

73. The attack rate of acute rheumatic fever after documented or
    proven streptococcal infections, in epidemic situations, is
    about ___ per cent:
    A. 10.0   D. 3.0
    B. 0.3   E. 15.0
    C. 5.8   Ref. 11 - p. 547

74. All of the following are associated with chickenpox, except:
    A. Incubation period 2-7 days
    B. Vesicular exanthem
    C. Attacks first face and back, then spreads downward
    D. Fever usually slight
    E. Slight leukocytosis   Ref. 11 - p. 670

75. The "sardonic grin" is associated with:
    A. Bell's palsy   D. Amyotonia congenita
    B. Rabies   E. Poliomyelitis
    C. Tetanus   Ref. 11 - p. 620

76. A 2 year-old child has a positive tuberculin reaction:
    A. No treatment is necessary
    B. Treat only if chest X-ray reveals pneumonia
    C. Treat with PASA 200 mg/day for 6 months
    D. Treat with streptomycin 1.0 gm/day for 1 month
    E. Treat with Isoniazid 10 to 20 mg/kg/day for one year
                                       Ref. 11 - pp. 635-636

77. Obstruction of the colon may be due to all, except:
    A. Carcinoma   D. Diverticulitis
    B. Adhesions   E. Hernia
    C. Volvulus   Ref. 4 - p. 955

78. When urgent operation for tetralogy of Fallot is required, the procedure should be:
    A. Open heart definitive reconstruction
    B. Pott's type anastomosis
    C. Blalock type anastomosis
    D. Direct aortic-pulmonary anastomosis
    E. Pulmonary artery banding   Ref. 6 - p. 724

79. The cyanotic child with congenital heart disease uses what mechanism to lessen exertional dyspnea?
    A. Squatting   D. Push-ups
    B. Deep breathing   E. Supine position
    C. Head down position   Ref. 6 - p. 681

80. Mediastinal lymphadenopathy causing respiratory distress may be due to:
    A. Tuberculosis   D. Lymphoma
    B. Sarcoidosis   E. All of the above
    C. Fungus infection   Ref. 6 - p. 663

81. The diagnosis of mucoviscidosis is established by:
    A. Sweat test for sodium loss
    B. Amylase in saliva
    C. Test of volume of sweat excretion
    D. Specific gravity of sputum
    E. Measurement of chromatids in sweat
        Ref. 6 - p. 634

82. Ulcerative colitis nearly always involves:
    A. Cecum   D. Left colon
    B. Right colon   E. Rectum
    C. Transverse colon   Ref. 4 - p. 973

83. In imperforate anus, immediate operation is not necessary if:
    A. There is a rectocutaneous or vaginal fistula
    B. The rectum is 2.5 cm above the perineum
    C. There is a rectovesical or urethral fistula
    D. Only a diaphragm exists
    E. The rectal pouch is high in the pelvis
        Ref. 6 - p. 1538

84. All of the following are early manifestations of congenital syphilis, except for:
    A. Paronychia and deformities of nails
    B. Dactylitis
    C. Saber shin
    D. Alopecia
    E. Rhinitis   Ref. 11 - p. 648

85. Which one of the following would be the last clinical manifestation of measles to appear:
    A. Low grade fever
    B. Koplik's spots
    C. Slight hacking cough
    D. Coryza
    E. Conjunctivitis
    Ref. 11 - pp. 654-655

86. Acute herpetic gingivostomatitis is not usually associated with:
    A. Symptoms usually insidious, appear slowly over period of weeks
    B. Fever often high (104 to 105 degrees F)
    C. Initial lesion is a vesicle which ruptures early
    D. Submaxillary lymphadenitis is common
    E. Lesions do not respond to antibiotic therapy
    Ref. 11 - p. 666

87. Variola major is characterized by all of the following, except:
    A. Incubation period usually 12 to 14 days
    B. Prodromal symptoms severe and start abruptly
    C. Fever is high and convulsions may occur
    D. Transient rashes during first two days are common
    E. Severity of symptoms increases as rash becomes papular
    Ref. 11 - pp. 673-674

88. Characteristic finding associated with acute infectious lymphocytosis:
    A. High white cell count (20,000 to 120,000 per mm^3)
    B. Lymphocytes abnormal: fragmented nuclei and vacuolated cytoplasm
    C. Marked eosinophilia (15 to 20%)
    D. Hypochromic, microcytic anemia
    E. Positive heterophil agglutination reaction
    Ref. 11 - pp. 693-694

89. ECHO virus has been associated with all of the following, except:
    A. Aseptic meningitis
    B. Acute glomerular nephritis
    C. Pleurodynia
    D. Myocarditis
    E. Maculopapular exanthems
    Ref. 11 - p. 712

90. Phycomycosis usually develops in association with:
    A. Uncontrolled diabetes
    B. Chronic diarrhea
    C. Burns
    D. All of the above
    E. None of the above
    Ref. 11 - p. 739

91. The operation of choice in ulcerative colitis with acute perforation is:
    A. Exteriorize the segment
    B. Total colectomy and ileostomy
    C. Close the perforation
    D. Proximal diverting colostomy
    E. Defunctionating ileostomy
    Ref. 6 - p. 1115

92. Systemic complications of ulcerative colitis include all, <u>except</u>:
    A. Carcinoma of the bile ducts   D. Peptic ulcer
    B. Arthralgias   E. Anemia
    C. Erythema nodosum   Ref. 4 - p. 976

93. The reason that the obstructed human appendix tends to rupture
    is that:
    A. It is a secreting organ
    B. Hypertonic contents attract fluid
    C. Bacteria incite exudation
    D. Any obstructed organ ruptures
    E. Fecaliths are chemically irritating
                                        Ref. 6 - p. 1168

94. Regional enteritis most commonly is misdiagnosed as:
    A. Small bowel obstruction   D. Perforated duodenal ulcer
    B. Acute appendicitis   E. Cancer of the cecum
    C. Ulcerative colitis   Ref. 6 - p. 1091

95. To be successful, the operation for duodenal ulcer must:
    A. Permanently control the acid factor
    B. Overcome any obstructive mechanism
    C. Remove surfaces which might bleed
    D. Leave a gastric pouch sufficient for physiologic needs
    E. All of the above   Ref. 6 - p. 1064

96. Cholecystectomy is advised for all patients with gallstones if
    they have a life expectancy of at least 6-8 years because:
    A. Serious complications increase in incidence with aging
    B. Concomitant diseases become more troublesome with age
    C. Operative mortality increases with each decade of delay
    D. Good operative results are jeopardized by advanced tissue
       changes
    E. All of the above are true   Ref. 6 - p. 1234

97. Patients in the "high risk group" for ulcerative colitis, who
    should be treated with surgery early in their course include all
    except:
    A. Children   D. Women 20-30 years of age
    B. Repeated severe attacks   E. Patients over 60 years of
    C. Total involvement of the colon   age
                                        Ref. 4 - p. 976

98. The chemotherapy for treating the larval stage of hydatid in-
    fections (echinococcosis):
    A. Hexylresorcinol   D. Antipar
    B. Diethylcarbamazine   E. None of the above
    C. Quinacrine   Ref. 11 - p. 765

99. All of the following are characteristic of necrotizing ulcerative gingivitis (Vincent's angina), except:
    A. Highly communicable infection, outbreaks common
    B. Fever, malaise and prominent fetid odor
    C. Gray necrotic membrane and small ulcers
    D. Painful hyperemic gingivae
    E. May be confused with herpetic stomatitis
    Ref. 11 - p. 799

100. Geographic tongue (wandering rash) should be treated with:
    A. Cleansing of mouth with oxidizing sprays
    B. Hourly rinses with half-strength hydrogen peroxide
    C. Topical steroids
    D. Penicillin (I. M.)
    E. None of the above   Ref. 11 - p. 801

101. Chemical changes in the serum associated with extensive and protracted vomiting in pyloric stenosis:
    A. Decrease in chloride concentration
    B. Increase in pH
    C. Increase in carbon dioxide content
    D. All of the above
    E. None of the above   Ref. 11 - p. 821

102. The lesions of granulomatous enterocolitis (Crohn's disease) are usually limited to the:
    A. Duodenum   D. Terminal ileum
    B. Proximal jejunum   E. Descending colon
    C. Proximal ileum   Ref. 11 - p. 837

103. Rectal and small bowel mucosae are apt to undergo avascular necrosis after doses of:
    A. 1, 500 r   D. 4, 500 r
    B. 2, 500 r   E. 5, 500 r
    C. 3, 500 r   Ref. 8 - pp. 278-283

104. Arsine used industrially is a cause of _____ poisoning:
    A. Arsenic   D. Carbon tetrachloride
    B. Lead   E. Cadmium
    C. Mercury   Ref. 2 - p. 57

105. The arthritis associated with hepatitis:
    A. Usually appears when the patient becomes icteric
    B. Has no relation to the appearance of icterus
    C. Usually disappears when the patient becomes icteric
    D. Causes deformity of the knee and ankle joints
    E. Is usually associated with hepatitis, type A
    Ref. 1 - p. 2005

106. "Mad as a hatter" refers to symptoms due to intoxication with:
A. Lead   D. Thallium
B. Arsenic   E. Antimony
C. Mercury   Ref. 2 - p. 61

107. A drug useful in removing resistant strains of meningococci from carriers is:
A. Streptomycin   D. Penicillin
B. Kanamycin   E. Sulfonamide
C. Amphotericin B   Ref. 2 - p. 335

108. In patients with rheumatic heart disease, continuous prophylaxis with antibiotics is most useful in the prevention of:
A. Congestive heart failure
B. Subacute bacterial endocarditis
C. Streptococcal pharyngitis
D. All of the above
E. None of the above   Ref. 2 - p. 306

109. The Rickettsial disease which is distinguished by the absence of a rash is:
A. Rickettsialpox   D. Flea-borne typhus fever
B. Q fever   E. Murine typhus
C. Rocky Mountain spotted fever Ref. 2 - p. 262

110. The usual symptoms in a case of acute inflammatory polyradiculoneuropathy include:
A. Abrupt onset of malaise D. Weakness which begins
B. Urinary retention   proximally
C. Unilateral distal weakness E. None of the above
           Ref. 2 - p. 787

111. Might also be found coexistent with chronic cervicitis:
A. Squamous metaplasia D. All of the above
B. Epidermidization   E. None of the above
C. Epidermoid hyperplasia Ref. 8 - pp. 234-237

112. Characteristics of pelvic tuberculosis include:
A. Accompanying pregnancy is rare
B. There is a high incidence of infertility
C. The tubercle bacillus will grow out of the menstrual blood in many instances
D. All of the above
E. None of the above   Ref. 8 - p. 424

113. Treatment of a pelvic abscess located in the cul-de-sac of Douglas:
A. Laparotomy   D. Posterior colpotomy
B. Antibiotics   E. Retroperitoneal drainage
C. Heparin   Ref. 8 - p. 397

114. A "chocolate cyst" of the ovary may be a:
   A. Endometrioma
   B. Corpus luteum hematoma
   C. Cystadenoma
   D. All of the above
   E. None of the above
   Ref. 8 - p. 545

115. The treatment for salpingitis isthmica nodosa is:
   A. Excisional biopsy
   B. Salpingectomy
   C. Antibiotics
   D. Douches and enzymes
   E. None of the above
   Ref. 8 - p. 411

116. Vulvar or vaginal tuberculosis:
   A. Has never been reported
   B. Has a neoplastic appearance
   C. May appear like a luetic lesion
   D. All of the above
   E. None of the above
   Ref. 8 - p. 421

117. On microscopic examination, tuberculous salpingitis may closely resemble:
   A. Lymphogranuloma
   B. Lues
   C. Adenocarcinoma
   D. None of the above
   E. All of the above
   Ref. 8 - p. 421

118. Heberden's nodes usually occur in:
   A. Rheumatoid arthritis
   B. Systemic lupus erythematosus
   C. Dermatomyositis
   D. Degenerative joint disease
   E. Charcot's joint
   Ref. 2 - p. 159

119. A case of Charcot-Marie-Tooth disease usually:
   A. Has exaggerated tendon reflexes in the lower extremities
   B. Has asymmetrical muscle weakness
   C. Has no sensory deficit demonstrable
   D. Has diminished lower extremity tendon reflexes
   E. None of the above
   Ref. 2 - p. 789

120. Hereditary acute intermittent porphyria is often mistaken for:
   A. Salicylate poisoning
   B. Phenobarbital poisoning
   C. Thallium poisoning
   D. Lead poisoning
   E. Arsenic poisoning
   Ref. 2 - p. 1874

121. Antimony compounds are used in the treatment of:
   A. Malaria
   B. Schistosomiasis
   C. Influenza
   D. Lymphogranuloma venereum
   E. Amebiasis
   Ref. 2 - p. 517

122. Which one of the following statements is true of Balkan nephritis?
   A. It is very rare in Yugoslavia
   B. It always occurs after pneumococcal infections
   C. Interstitial fibrosis is very prominent
   D. The primary lesion involves the glomeruli
   E. Tetracycline is the treatment of choice
   Ref. 2 - p. 1154

123. Complications of renal transplantation may include:
    A. Ureteric fistula
    B. "Transplant lung"
    C. Hypertension
    D. All of the above
    E. None of the above
    Ref. 2 - p. 1117

124. Renal transplantation is most likely to be successful if the donor is:
    A. An unrelated cadaver
    B. Of the same blood group
    C. An identical twin
    D. The mother
    E. The father
    Ref. 2 - p. 1116

125. Dysfunctional uterine bleeding may include bleeding due to:
    A. Fibroids
    B. Endocervical polyp
    C. Irregular endometrial shedding
    D. Granulosa cell tumor
    E. None of the above
    Ref. 8 - p. 692

126. Characteristics of dysmenorrhea due to endometriosis include:
    A. It gets worse after the flow begins
    B. It is usually relieved by cervical dilatation
    C. It is most frequently seen in women in their late 30's
    D. The pain may not be in proportion to the amount of disease present
    Ref. 8 - pp. 559-560

127. In a 38-year-old woman with extensive pelvic endometriosis, the treatment of choice is:
    A. Estrogen - progesterone suppression of ovulation
    B. Excision of endometrial implants
    C. Progesterone treatment
    D. Hysterectomy
    E. Hysterectomy and bilateral salpingo-oophorectomy
    Ref. 8 - p. 560

128. In a patient treated for choriocarcinoma, conception:
    A. Should be undertaken immediately
    B. Can never occur because patients are rendered sterile after treatment
    C. May be undertaken after one year if HCG titers are negative
    D. None of the above
    Ref. 8 - p. 612

129. _____ is employed to measure ovarian follicular maturation during pergonal (HMG) therapy.
    A. Serum LH
    B. Serum FSH
    C. Serum progesterone
    D. 24 hour urine for pregnanediol
    E. 24 hour urine for estrogen
    Ref. 8 - p. 654

130. Which is pathognomonic of abdominal pregnancy?
    A. Eccentric position of the fetus
    B. Lack of outline of the uterine wall
    C. Fetal parts are easily palpable
    D. Fetal parts appear lateral to the lumbar spine on a lateral
       X-ray
    E. None of the above   Ref. 9 - p. 186

131. In spontaneous rupture of the membranes:
    A. The cause is unknown
    B. If it occurs prior to 35 weeks one should await fetal maturity
    C. Induce labor within 24-48 hours if it occurs past 37 weeks
    D. All of the above
    E. None of the above   Ref. 9 - p. 363

132. The cell type used in the histocompatibility tests for renal
    transplantation is:
    A. Red blood cell   D. Plasma cell
    B. Leukocyte   E. All of the above
    C. Mast cell   Ref. 2 - p. 1116

133. Viokase is used in the treatment of:
    A. Pancreatic insufficiency   D. Hepatitis
    B. Biliary colic   E. Carcinoma of the colon
    C. Duodenal ulcer   Ref. 2 - p. 1229

134. In acute pancreatitis, the serum amylase usually becomes
    elevated approximately _____ after the onset of illness:
    A. 1-2 hours   D. 48-72 hours
    B. 3-6 hours   E. 2-5 days
    C. 24-48 hours   Ref. 2 - p. 1246

135. A deficiency of jejunal lactase usually leads to diarrhea follow-
    ing ingestion of:
    A. Milk   D. Fish
    B. Bananas   E. Gluten-containing bread
    C. Peanuts   Ref. 2 - p. 1232

136. Which of the following is a fat-soluble vitamin?
    A. Vitamin A   D. Vitamin C
    B. Vitamin B_2 E. Folic acid
    C. Vitamin B_{12} Ref. 2 - p. 1222

137. Macrophages with positive periodic acid-Schiff-staining ma-
    terial in lymph nodes are characteristically found in:
    A. Wilson's disease   D. Peutz-Jeghers syndrome
    B. Hodgkin's disease   E. Gardner's syndrome
    C. Whipple's disease   Ref. 2 - p. 1235

138. The normal 24 hour urinary excretion of D-xylose after a
25 gram oral dose is:
A. Greater than 5 mg   D. Greater than 15 grams
B. Greater than 500 mg   E. Greater than 1 gram
C. Greater than 5 grams   Ref. 2 - p. 1224

139. The usual manner of death from eclampsia is:
A. During and as a result of continued convulsions
B. Congestive heart failure
C. Cardiac arrest during a convulsion
D. Uremia
E. Hemorrhagic bronchopneumonia Ref. 9 - p. 314

140. _____ is the most common malignancy to metastasize to the
placenta and/or fetus.
A. Hodgkin's disease   D. Adenocarcinoma of the
B. Breast carcinoma   endometrium
C. Osteosarcoma   E. Malignant melanoma
                                 Ref. 7 - p. 818

141. The incidence of puerperal thrombophlebitis is decreased be-
cause:
A. Deliveries are less traumatic
B. Of asepsis
C. Of early ambulation
D. All of the above
E. None of the above   Ref. 9 - p. 496

142. Following delivery, ureteral dilatation (of pregnancy) resolves
in _____ weeks.
A. 1   D. 6
B. 2   E. 8
C. 4   Ref. 7 - p. 752

143. Recurrent pulmonary emboli from pelvic thrombophlebitis is
best treated with:
A. Anticoagulants
B. Ligation of femoral veins
C. Ligation of inferior vena cava
D. Paravertebral block of sympathetic chain
E. Ligation of inferior vena cava and ovarian veins
                                 Ref. 9 - p. 496

144. The pinard maneuver is seen:
A. In low cervical sections
B. In forceps rotation maneuvers
C. In breech deliveries
D. As an adjunct to version and extraction
E. None of the above   Ref. 7 - p. 1154

145. Concerning fetal heart tones:
    A. The rate is of no clinical significance
    B. A rate of over 150 is abnormal
    C. A rate under 120 is abnormal
    D. Irregularity is a sign of distress
    E. None of the above   Ref. 9 - p. 396

146. The measurement of urinary forminoglutamic acid (FIGLU) is used to demonstrate deficiency of:
    A. Iron   D. Riboflavin
    B. Folic acid   E. Niacin
    C. Vitamin B_{12} Ref. 2 - p. 1410

147. The usual manifestations of salmonella typhosum infection may include:
    A. Headache   D. All of the above
    B. Relative bradycardia   E. None of the above
    C. Frequent splenomegaly   Ref. 1 - p. 804

148. The incidence of monilia infections is increased most often in patients with:
    A. Thyrotoxicosis   D. Acromegaly
    B. Hyperparathyroidism   E. XXY syndrome
    C. Hypoparathyroidism   Ref. 1 - p. 903

149. Which one of the following statements regarding gonococcus is true?
    A. It is a gram positive bacillus
    B. It may produce endocarditis
    C. Efficient artificial immunization is available against gono-coccal infections
    D. It is always associated with syphilitic infection
    E. Tetracycline is generally useless in the treatment of infec-tions due to this organism   Ref. 1 - p. 790

150. Myasthenia gravis is associated with _____ in a large percent-age of cases:
    A. Syphilis   D. Systemic lupus erythema-
    B. Thymoma   tosus
    C. Sarcoidosis   E. Thyroid adenomas
                                   Ref. 2 - p. 802

151. Which one of the following drugs is not useful in the treatment of pulmonary tuberculosis?
    A. Cycloserine   D. Paromomycin
    B. Streptomycin   E. Pyrazinamide
    C. Ethionamide   Ref. 1 - p. 867

152. High forceps operations _____ :
    A. Occur when application is made to an unengaged head
    B. Are relatively common in practice
    C. Are the procedure of choice in acute fetal distress
    D. Are usually atraumatic
    E. Are best done with Piper's Forceps
                                    Ref. 7 - p. 1120

153. The most common cause of perinatal morbidity and mortality is:
    A. Obstetrical trauma   D. Toxemia
    B. Sepsis   E. Prematurity
    C. Hemorrhage   Ref. 7 - p. 526

154. Microscopically is often mistaken for adenomyosis of fallopian tube:
    A. Follicular salpingitis   D. Tuberculous salpingitis
    B. Hydrosalpinx simplex   E. None of the above
    C. Salpingitis isthmica nodosa   Ref. 8 - p. 411

155. The pelvic axis (curve of carus):
    A. Is an imaginary line which passes through the center of any pelvic plane
    B. Is the plane of greatest pelvic dimension
    C. Is the plane of least pelvic dimension
    D. Is the same as pelvic inclination
    E. Is parallel to the pelvic outlet   Ref. 7 - p. 296

156. The female external genitalia develop embryologically from the:
    A. Urogenital sinus   D. Genital eminence
    B. Genital swellings   E. None of the above
    C. Genital tubercle   Ref. 8 - p. 134

157. The epoophoron are:
    A. Unfused portions of the Mullarian ducts
    B. Vestigual structures of the urogenital sinus
    C. Remants of Wolffian ducts
    D. Urogenital ridges
    E. None of the above   Ref. 8 - p. 132

158. Complications of Paget's disease may include:
    A. High output cardiac failure   D. All of the above
    B. Fractures   E. None of the above
    C. Sarcoma development   Ref. 1 - p. 1975

159. Each of the following statements regarding cholera is true, except:
    A. The organisms produce an exotoxin
    B. Hypovolemic shock is common
    C. Metabolic alkalosis is common
    D. Serious hypokalamia can occur
    E. The carrier state occurs in about 4% of convalescent patients
                                    Ref. 1 - p. 856

160. Reduced blood volume incident to bleeding shows all, <u>except</u>:
   A. Rise in central venous pressure
   B. Stimulation of baroreceptor tone
   C. Fall in cardiac output
   D. Initiation of sympatho-adrenal response
   E. Increase in peripheral resistance by vasoconstriction
   Ref. 6 - p. 134

161. The left ventricular end-diastolic pressure may be commonly
   elevated in each of the following, <u>except</u>:
   A. Left ventricular failure   D. Constrictive pericarditis
   B. Early mitral stenosis   E. Restrictive myocardial
   C. Aortic incompetence   disease
   Ref. 1 - p. 1185

162. Following resection of two-thirds of the liver, complete re-
   generation occurs in:
   A. 2-3 weeks   D. 2-3 months
   B. 4-6 weeks   E. 4-6 months
   C. 6-8 weeks   Ref. 4 - p. 1013

163. Macrocytic anemia may be due to each of the following, <u>except</u>:
   A. Liver disease   D. Antimetabolite therapy
   B. Hypothyroidism   E. Intestinal malabsorption
   C. Iron deficiency   Ref. 1 - p. 1583

164. All of the following are unconjugated hyperbilirubinemias,
   except for:
   A. Transient neonatal hyperbilirubinemia
   B. Crigler-Najjar syndrome
   C. Dubin-Johnson syndrome
   D. Gilbert's syndrome
   E. Hemolysis due to maternal-fetal blood group incompatibili-
      ties   Ref. 11 - p. 879

165. The normal portal pressure is less than:
   A. 50-100 mm H₂O   D. 350-400 mm H₂O
   B. 100-200 mm H₂O   E. 400-500 mm H₂O
   C. 250-300 mm H₂O   Ref. 6 - p. 1197

166. All of the following are true about the female urethra, <u>except</u>:
   A. Is entirely lined by transitional epithelium
   B. Skene's ducts open into the lower border of the meatus
   C. Has an inner longitudinal and outer circular layer of muscu-
      lature
   D. Caruncle is the most common benign tumor of the urethra
   E. Carcinoma of the urethra is rare
   Ref. 8 - p. 3

167. Urinary incontinence results from all of the following, except:
    A. Ectopic ureter
    B. Vesicovaginal fistula
    C. Rectovesical fistula
    D. Neurogenic bladder
    E. Bladder infection
    Ref. 6 - p. 1550

168. Each of the following principles regarding the treatment of infections in renal failure is usually true, except:
    A. Strenuous efforts should be made to identify the causative organisms before starting antimicrobial therapy
    B. Narrow-spectrum antimicrobials should be employed whenever possible
    C. The loading dose of antimicrobials must be reduced at least four fold
    D. The size of the maintenance doses must be adjusted to renal function
    E. Spacing of the maintenance doses must be adjusted to renal function
    Ref. 2 - p. 1104

169. In patients with cholangitis and common duct obstruction, each of the following is commonly elevated in serum, except:
    A. Alkaline phosphatase
    B. 5-nucleotidase
    C. Leucine-aminopeptidase
    D. SGOT
    E. Albumin
    Ref. 2 - p. 1317

170. The BSP (bromsulphalein) test is not valid in the presence of any of the following except:
    A. Hepatic dysfunction of any degree
    B. Bilirubin greater than 5 mg %
    C. Obstruction of the bile ducts
    D. Obesity
    E. High fever
    Ref. 4 - p. 1015

171. Common causes of alveolar hypoventilation may include each of the following, except:
    A. Obstruction to the airways
    B. Damage to the medullary centers by disease
    C. Early diabetic acidosis
    D. Injury to the chest wall
    E. Paralysis of the musculature of the thorax
    Ref. 1 - p. 546

172. In regard to bone healing, the following are correct, except:
    A. The initial acid reaction at fracture site keeps Ca in solution till needed
    B. The hematoma around fracture fragment ends inhibits bone healing
    C. Bone cells become active in 10-14 days when reaction becomes alkaline
    D. New bone comes in part from metaplasia of fibroblasts
    E. Inflammatory stiffening of tissues at fracture site is a natural splinting
    Ref. 4 - p. 1328

173. Each of the following statements regarding disordered hemostasis due to disorders of vessels and platelets is true, except:
    A. Petechiae are common
    B. A positive family history is rarely obtained
    C. Hemarthroses are characteristic
    D. Bleeding often occurs immediately following trauma
    E. Females are afflicted more commonly than males
    Ref. 1 - pp. 1648, 1655

174. The symptoms of endemic goiter include all of the following, except:
    A. Cold intolerance
    B. Heat intolerance
    C. Hoarseness
    D. Dysphagia
    E. Enlargement of the thyroid gland
    Ref. 2 - p. 1726

175. Regarding the kidneys, all of the following statements are true, except:
    A. Renal arteries originate from the aorta at 2nd lumbar level
    B. Each renal artery branch is an end artery
    C. The left renal artery is longer than the right
    D. The capsular lymphatics drain into infradiaphragmatic periaortic nodes
    E. The left renal vein receives adrenal and gonadal blood
    Ref. 6 - p. 1547

176. All are seen in thrombophlebitis of an extremity, except:
    A. Mild systemic manifestations of fever and tachycardia
    B. Sensation of heaviness of leg
    C. Unilateral increase in the circumference
    D. Increased skin heat
    E. Follmer''s sign
    Ref. 7 - p. 1101

177. Causes of death in patients with cirrhosis and varices include all, except:
    A. Hemorrhage
    B. Hepatic failure
    C. Renal shut-down
    D. Infection
    E. Myocardial infarction
    Ref. 4 - p. 1025

178. The liver performs all of the following functions, except:
    A. Stores, converts and de-aminates amino acids
    B. Forms vitamin A and stores A, D and B_{12}
    C. Forms erythrocytes in the adult
    D. Breaks down hemoglobin and forms bile salts, acids and pigments
    E. Forms plasma albumins, globulins and fibrinogen
    Ref. 6 - p. 1178

179. The usual drug used to treat the Eaton-Lambert syndrome is:
    A. Vincristine
    B. Guanidine
    C. Chlorambucil
    D. Vinblastine
    E. 6-mercaptopurine
    Ref. 2 - p. 805

180. Complications of acute cholecystitis include each of the following, except:
A. Pancreatitis
B. Peritonitis
C. Biliary fistula
D. Perforation
E. Migratory thrombophlebitis
Ref. 2 - p. 1316

181. Unless the cause of acute pancreatitis is corrected, all of the following may develop over a period of time, except:
A. Intraductal stone formation
B. Beta cell adenoma
C. Pseudocyst
D. Chronic fibrosis
E. Diffuse calcification
Ref. 6 - p. 1263

182. Each of the following drugs may be useful in "resistant cases" of tuberculosis, except:
A. Ethambutol
B. Penicillin
C. Viomycin
D. Pyrazinamide
E. Cycloserine
Ref. 1 - p. 868

183. Superior vena caval obstruction shows itself by all, except:
A. Prominent veins over upper chest
B. Edema of head, neck and arms
C. Dry conjunctivas from decreased tear formation
D. Distended neck veins
E. Ruddy cyanosis of head, neck and upper chest
Ref. 6 - p. 662

184. Each of the following findings may be consistent with left ventricular hypertrophy, except;
A. A mean QRS axis of $180°$ in the frontal plane
B. An R wave measuring more than 20 mm in Lead I
C. An S wave measuring more than 25 mm in Lead V_1
D. An R wave measuring more than 25 mm in Lead V_6
E. A mean QRS axis of $-15°$ in the frontal plane
Ref. 1 - p. 1090

185. Causes of neutropenia may include each of the following, except:
A. Polycythemia vera
B. Typhoid fever
C. Felty's syndrome
D. Aplastic anemia
E. Acute lymphatic leukemia
Ref. 1 - p. 317

186. The following statements about burns are correct, except:
A. Narcotics and other drugs should be given intravenously in the early stages
B. Burns of over 50% of body surface should have fluids calculated as for 50% burn in order to avoid overloading
C. Children and old persons should receive less than calculated amounts of fluid
D. Respiratory tract burns require maximal limitation of fluid
E. The exposure method is especially indicated in circumferential burns
Ref. 6 - p. 253

187. All of the following are characteristic of congenital aortic stenosis, except:
   A. Accounts for 3% of all cardiac manifestations
   B. Stenosis is valvular, leaflets thickened
   C. Child usually symptomatic with poor physical development
   D. Heart size usually normal
   E. If gradient of pressure across aortic valve is small, then EKG is normal   Ref. 11 - pp. 1064-1065

188. The following statements about thyroid hyperplasia are correct, except:
   A. Papillary infolding of acini is due to crowding of the new cells
   B. Nodule formation is due to uneven distribution of hyperplasia
   C. Colloid-empty follicles are caused by increased secretory rate
   D. Increased blood flow is evidenced by bruit and thrill over the thyroid
   E. The accompanying lymphoid hyperplasia is an unexplained phenomenon   Ref. 6 - p. 1446

Each group of questions below consists of lettered headings followed by a list of numbered words or phrases. For each numbered word or phrase select the one heading which is most closely related to it:

   A. Argentaffin cells
   B. Myenteric ganglion cells in distal colon
   C. Myenteric (Auerbach's) plexus
   D. Webs of the mucosa
   E. Parietal cells

189. ___ Achalasia
190. ___ Carcinoid syndrome
191. ___ Plummer-Vinson syndrome
192. ___ Hirschsprung's disease
193. ___ Peptic ulcer   Ref. 2 - pp. 1181, 1795,
                                          1179, 1193,
                                          1200

Match item with pneumothorax treatment:

   A. No therapy needed
   B. Water seal drainage
   C. Thoracotomy

194. ___ Over 25% pneumothorax
195. ___ Multiple blebs of lung
196. ___ Asymptomatic, under 25%
197. ___ Recurrent case
198. ___ Tension pneumothorax   Ref. 6 - p. 612

A. Hypophosphatasia
B. Familial dysautonomia
C. Osteopetrosis
D. Cleidocranial dysostosis
E. Ectodermal dysplasia

199. ___ Small and malformed teeth, union of midportion of upper lip to the anterior maxillary gingival tissue
200. ___ Recessive transmitted condition, irregular and incomplete bone formation, teeth small with abnormal roots
201. ___ Disorder of bone arising during fetal life, basilar skull and orbits affected, peculiar facies, hypoplastic mandible
202. ___ Complete or almost complete anodontia, body of maxilla is underdeveloped
203. ___ Abnormal chewing and swallowing, severe vomiting attacks, insensitivity to pain, tooth grinding, aberrant behavioral and speech patterns   Ref. 10 - p. 1865

Match the following:

A. Squamous lung carcinoma
B. Alveolar cell carcinoma
C. Oat cell carcinoma
D. Adenocarcinoma
E. Carcinoid

204. ___ Secretes ACTH
205. ___ Also known as scar carcinoma
206. ___ Most common lung carcinoma
207. ___ Secretes ADH
208. ___ Bronchial adenoma   Ref. 4 - p. 1848, 1853

A. Infantile eczema
B. Flexural eczema
C. Dyshidrotic eczema
D. Nummular eczema
E. Generalized atopic dermatitis

209. ___ Found on cheeks, neck creases, ears and scalp, cheeks are rosy, exudative, moist, papular
210. ___ Found on palms and soles, intensely pruritic, blisters
211. ___ Occurs usually after age 4 years, sides of neck, erythema, excoriation, skin become lichenified and taut
212. ___ Uncommon in young children, hands and feet cold, eyelids are lichenified , intraorbital pigmentation
213. ___ Found on extremities and trunk, circular, papulovesicular patches, often pruritic, lesions sparse or numerous
          Ref. 10 - p. 1807

A. Idiopathic alveolar hypoventilation
B. Pickwickian syndrome
C. Bronchiectasis
D. Chronic bronchitis
E. Ankylosing spondylitis

214. ___ Normal total lung capacity, with decrease in vital capacity and maximal breathing capacity
215. ___ Raised PCO_2, with arterial desaturation in a patient with normal pulmonary and thoracic cage mechanics
216. ___ Raised PCO_2 with arterial desaturation in an obese patient
217. ___ May result as a complication of mucoviscidosis
218. ___ Mucous gland hyperplasia and productive cough

Ref. 2 - pp. 818-824

Match cause and effect in response to injury:

A. Antidiuretic hormone release
B. Catecholamine secretion
C. Mobilization of bone Ca and P
D. ACTH release
E. Chemical inflammation

219. ___ Afferent nerve stimuli from injured area
220. ___ Hypovolemic shock
221. ___ Chemically active secretions in peritoneum
222. ___ Bacterial endotoxin
223. ___ Body immobilization

Ref. 6 - p. 2

A. Diphtheria
B. Scarlet fever
C. Measles
D. Chickenpox
E. Poliomyelitis

224. ___ Child may return to school 5 days after appearance of rash, immune contacts may re-enter school without restriction
225. ___ Return to school after 2-3 negative nose and throat cultures
226. ___ Return to school no less than 7 days from onset of illness, immune contacts may re-enter school without restriction
227. ___ Return to school when crusts have formed
228. ___ Return to school one week after onset of symptoms or after defervescence, whichever is longer

Ref. 11 - p. 568

Match type of urinary calculus with appearance:

A. Calcium oxalate
B. Triple phosphate
C. Uric acid
D. Cystine
E. Foreign body

229. ___ Yellow, orange or pink
230. ___ Encrusted appearance
231. ___ Dark colored with sharp spicules
232. ___ "Maple sugar"
233. ___ Porous, soft, tan or white   Ref. 6 - p. 1561

A. Urokinase
B. Arvin
C. Dipyridamole
D. Coumarin
E. Heparin

234. ___ Activates the fibrinolytic system
235. ___ Experimentally used defibrinating agent
236. ___ Main effect is on vitamin K dependent factors
237. ___ Protamine counteracts effects
238. ___ Inhibits platelet functions   Ref. 2 - pp. 912, 914, 915

A. Inappropriate secretion of ADH
B. Anion gap
C. Metabolic alkalosis
D. Hypokalemia
E. Hypomagnesemia

239. ___ Increase in lactic acidosis
240. ___ Bicarbonate concentration that is increased without an
equivalent increase in the PCO_2
241. ___ Masked by diabetic acidosis
242. ___ Dilutional hyponatremia, normal BUN, and absence of edema
243. ___ Often develops in malabsorption syndromes

Ref. 1 - pp. 1347, 1356,
1358, 1364,
1366

Match the following:

A. Ligamentum venosum
B. Ligamentum teres
C. Hypogastric ligaments
D. Patent ductus
E. Urachus

244. ___ Ductus venosus
245. ___ Umbilical vein

246. ___ Umbilical artery
247. ___ Yolk sac
248. ___ Ductus arterium   Ref. 7 - pp. 211-215

Match motor function loss with appropriate nerve:

A. Ulnar
B. Median
C. Radial

249. ___ Inability to spread fingers
250. ___ Inability to extend wrist
251. ___ Inability to oppose all finger tips
252. ___ Inability to make a fist
253. ___ Inability to oppose thumb and little finger
                                        Ref. 6 - p. 1906

A. Graves' disease
B. Thyrotoxicosis factitia
C. Both
D. Neither

254. ___ Infiltrative ophthalmopathy
255. ___ Low BMR
256. ___ Low 24 hour ^{131}I uptake by the thyroid gland
257. ___ High cholesterol
258. ___ High T_3-resin uptake   Ref. 1 - pp. 475,477

A. Cyanosis
B. Pulmonary hypertension
C. Both
D. Neither

259. ___ Patent ductus arteriosus
260. ___ Ventricular septal defect
261. ___ Tetralogy of Fallot
262. ___ Coarctation of aorta
263. ___ Transposition of great vessels   Ref. 6 - p. 677

A. Pulmonary stenosis
B. Mitral valvular stenosis
C. Both
D. Neither

264. ___ May be congenital
265. ___ Heart failure may occur
266. ___ May resemble hemodynamic features of left atrial myxoma
267. ___ An opening "snap" may be present
268. ___ Straightening of the left border of the cardiac silhouette
         typically occurs   Ref. 1 - pp. 1184,1162

Match the following:

A. ASD
B. VSD
C. Both
D. Neither

269. ___ Often close spontaneously
270. ___ Commonly leads to pulmonary hypertension
271. ___ Most common congenital cardiac lesion
272. ___ Left-to-right shunt
273. ___ Should be closed surgically   Ref. 4 - pp. 1951-1979

A. Infectious hepatitis
B. Serum hepatitis
C. Both
D. Neither

274. ___ Prolonged viremia for years
275. ___ Spread by mosquito bites
276. ___ Incubation period 7-10 days
277. ___ Case fatality rate very low
278. ___ Protection afforded by immune globulin
                                          Ref. 10 - p. 707

A. Massive pulmonary infarction
B. Lobar pneumonia
C. Both
D. Neither

279. ___ Herpes labialis
280. ___ Hemoptysis
281. ___ Normal lung scan
282. ___ Chest pain
283. ___ Diagnosis is often made by pulmonary angiogram
                          Ref. 2 - pp. 283, 281, 918,
                                                919

A. Fracture site hematoma
B. Soft tissue hematoma
C. Both
D. Neither

284. ___ Should be removed by aspiration or incision
285. ___ Essential to proper healing
286. ___ Is invaded by inflammatory cells
287. ___ Tends to calcify
288. ___ Has high level of acid phosphatase
                                    Ref. 4 - p. 1328

A. Rickettsialpox
B. Rocky Mountain spotted fever
C. Both
D. Neither

289. ___ Body louse is the arthropod vector
290. ___ Cattle are the animal reservoirs
291. ___ Cutaneous rash spreads centrally, involves palms and soles
292. ___ Untreated mortality 10-40%
293. ___ Complement fixation specific   Ref. 11 - p. 730

A. Staphylococcus
B. Streptococcus
C. Both
D. Neither

294. ___ Koplik's spots
295. ___ Subacute bacterial endocarditis
296. ___ Scarlet fever
297. ___ Pneumonia
298. ___ Vincent's angina   Ref. 1 - pp. 772,778

A. Pernicious anemia
B. Chloramphenicol
C. Pure red cell aplasia
D. Sideroblastic anemia
E. Paroxysmal nocturnal hemoglobinuria

299. ___ Impairment of mitochondrial protein synthesis, with vacuolated erythroid precursors in the marrow
300. ___ Associated with antibodies directed against erythroid precursors
301. ___ DNA synthesis greatly impaired, with relatively normal RNA synthesis
302. ___ Impairment of normal incorporation of iron into porphyrin
303. ___ Markedly low leukocyte alkaline phosphatase
          Ref. 2 - pp. 1405, 1418, 1419, 1424, 1437

A. Syncytial cells of placenta
B. Cytotrophoblastic cells of placenta (Langhans cells)
C. Both
D. Neither

304. ___ Rich in cytoplasmic RNA
305. ___ Responsible for synthesis of chorionic gonadotrophin
306. ___ Secretes placental steroid hormones
307. ___ Involved in pinocytosis
308. ___ Begin to thin out at about 17-18 weeks of pregnancy
          Ref. 9 - pp. 115-116

After each of the following case histories there is a series of
multiple choice questions based on the history. Select the one
most appropriate answer:

CASE (Questions 309-312): A 21 year-old multipara delivers a ma-
cerated fetus which has been dead for 10 weeks. After delivery she
continues to bleed.

309. The most likely etiology of a maternal hemorrhagic diathesis
     in a woman with an intrauterine fetal demise occurring five or
     more weeks previously is:
     A. Vitamin K deficiency   D. Hypoplasminogenemia
     B. Factor V deficiency   E. All of the above
     C. Hypofibrinogenemia   Ref. 7 - pp. 1007-1008

310. What is the usual presentation of an anencephalic fetus?
     A. Cephalic   D. Compound presentation
     B. Breech   E. None of the above
     C. Transverse lie   Ref. 7 - p. 325

311. Hydramnios accompanies anencephaly in approximately
     _____ % of cases:
     A. 20%   D. 90%
     B. 50%   E. 100%
     C. 70%   Ref. 7 - p. 1071

312. Characteristics of anencephalics include:
     A. Low maternal estriol secretion
     B. Fetal adrenal hypoplasia
     C. Late onset of labor after 42 weeks
     D. All
     E. A and C only   Ref. 7 - pp. 1071-1072

CASE (Questions 313-316): A 35 year-old male was seen because of
a history of frequent headaches. The blood pressure in both upper
limbs was 180/100 mm Hg. In the lower limbs the blood pressure
was 120/70 mm Hg. There was a systolic bruit heard in the left
interscapular area.

313. The most probable diagnosis is:
     A. Aortic incompetence   D. Coarctation of the aorta
     B. Essential hypertension   E. Pheochromocytoma
     C. Patent ductus arteriosus

314. An X-ray of the chest is most likely to reveal:
 A. Straightening of the left border of the heart
 B. Prominent pulmonary vascular markings
 C. Notching of the ribs
 D. Dumb-bell tumor
 E. Giant left atrium

315. This condition is seen most often in patients with:
 A. Familial hyperlipoproteinemia
 B. Turner's syndrome
 C. Syphilitic aortitis
 D. Rheumatic heart disease
 E. Klinefelter's syndrome

316. The treatment of choice for this disorder is usually:
 A. Valve prosthesis
 B. Low salt diet
 C. Adrenalectomy
 D. Aortic prosthesis
 E. Ligation of the ductus arteriosus

Ref. 2 - p. 941

CASE (Questions 317-320): A 40 year-old housewife has been complaining of joint pains in both hands intermittently for five years. During the past year she has been feeling very weak, anorectic, and has lost about 20 pounds. She states that all the joints in the hands feel stiff in the morning but the stiffness gradually disappears as the day progresses. The joints on examination were swollen. Tenderness was elicited on pressure and on passive motion of the joints. There was ulnar deviation of both hands. There was no history of Raynaud's phenomenon elicited. She had a temperature of 101° F. Apart from these joint complaints and the mild systemic symptoms, her past history was completely negative.

317. Which one of the following abnormalities is found most commonly in her illness?
 A. A diastolic cardiac murmur
 B. Hypocalcemia
 C. High titres of rheumatoid factor
 D. Hyperuricemia
 E. Cirrhosis of the liver

318. A long-term renal complication of her illness may be:
 A. Recurrent kidney stones
 B. Renal amyloidosis
 C. Kimmelsteil-Wilson kidney
 D. Hepato-renal syndrome
 E. Flea-bitten kidney

319. The agent most useful in her management probably is:
 A. Aspirin
 B. Methotrexate
 C. Allopurinol
 D. Digitalis
 E. B-complex vitamins

320. Pneumoconiosis associated with pulmonary manifestations of this illness is known as:
    A. Idiopathic hemosiderosis
    B. Caplan's syndrome
    C. Middle lobe syndrome
    D. "Senile lung" syndrome
    E. Hypertrophic pulmonary osteoarthropathy
    Ref. 2 - pp. 144-146

CASE (Questions 321-324): An 18 year-old girl had sudden pain in the left chest with cough, fever and wheezing on respiration. The x-ray suggested pneumonia. After antibiotics had been started, she experienced brisk hemoptysis.

321. Diagnosis at this time will be made by:
    A. X-ray tomogram
    B. Bronchoscopy and bronchogram
    C. Typing sputum for pneumococcus
    D. Specific response to antibiotics
    E. Bronchoscopic biopsy if a smooth tumor is seen

322. On bronchoscopy, a smooth, round tumor is seen partially obstructing the left main bronchus. Which statement is false?
    A. This is a bronchial adenoma, probably benign
    B. Endobronchial excision is risky because of dumbbell extension
    C. Endobronchial biopsy is done at this time
    D. This may be a carcinoid type of tumor
    E. Thoracotomy is indicated

323. What influences decision as to approach and procedure?
    A. Contraindications to thoracotomy mandate bronchoscopic treatment
    B. Degenerative lung changes distal to bronchial obstruction
    C. Wide extension outside the bronchial wall
    D. Active infection in lung or pleura
    E. All of the above

324. At thoracotomy, since the left main bronchus is involved:
    A. Only pneumonectomy is technically possible
    B. Biopsy for diagnosis and then close for X-ray therapy
    C. Do a lobectomy, no matter what the lung status
    D. Bronchotomy, tumor removal and plastic closure is advised
    E. Shave off the tumor flush with bronchial wall to overcome obstruction
    Ref. 6 - pp. 643-644

CASE (Questions 325-328): A 42 year-old woman is admitted to the hospital with a large lesion of the cervix which on biopsy was interpreted as invasive squamous cell carcinoma. On pelvic exam the cancer was felt to extend beyond the cervix but not to the lateral pelvic wall and did not involve the bladder, rectum or lower third of the vagina

325. The international classification of this lesion is:
    A. Stage IV   D. Stage I
    B. Stage III   E. Stage O
    C. Stage II   Ref. 8 - p. 275

326. The most suitable treatment would be:
    A. Anterior exenteration   D. Hormones
    B. Posterior exenteration   E. Abdominal hysterectomy
    C. Irradiation   Ref. 8 - p. 277

327. The overall 5 year survival rate with the preceding therapy is:
    A. 30%   D. 60%
    B. 40%   E. 70%
    C. 50%   Ref. 8 - p. 277

328. The stage of the disease is more important than the cell type
    from the standpoint of:
    A. Radiosensitivity   D. Type of irradiation used
    B. Prognosis   E. None of the above
    C. Radioresistance   Ref. 8 - pp. 248, 277

CASE (Questions 329-332): A 40 year-old man complained of severe
pain in the precordium following an emotional upset. The pain
radiated to the left mandible. The patient was given some pills to
take sublingually and the pain disappeared in about three minutes.
A physical examination and EKG taken after the attack of pain were
normal.

329. The most probable etiology of his chest pain is:
    A. Acute myocardial infarction D. Neurocirculatory asthenia
    B. Angina pectoris   E. Pulmonary infarction
    C. Teitze syndrome

330. The pills which relieved his pain probably were:
    A. Aminophylline   D. Prednisone
    B. Nitroglycerine   E. Aspirin
    C. Digoxin

331. An abnormality in the EKG is most likely to occur during:
    A. Sleep   D. Early morning
    B. Immediately before eating E. Late evening
    C. An attack of chest pain

332. The most common cause of this ailment is:
    A. Aortic stenosis
    B. Aortic regurgitation
    C. Syphilis
    D. Atherosclerosis of coronary vessels
    E. Aneurysm of the sinus of valsalva
                              Ref. 2 - p. 994

CASE (Questions 333-336): A 35 year-old male had been having intermittent diplopia and tremor of the right arm, occasionally associated
with ataxia. Between these episodes he was asymptomatic. Recently
he had been complaining of incontinence and marked weakness in both
lower limbs. There was no appreciable muscle wasting in the lower
limbs. The deep tendon reflexes in the lower extremities were exaggerated but were normal in the upper extremities. No sensory
deficits were noted. There were no other abnormal findings on
neurological examination.

333. The most probable diagnosis is:
   A. Guillain-Barré syndrome   D. Brain abscess
   B. Spinal cord tumor   E. Multiple sclerosis
   C. Herpes simplex encephalitis

334. This illness is:
   A. Three times more common in men than in women
   B. Three times more common in women than in men
   C. Equally common in both sexes
   D. Usually preceded by exposure to venereal diseases
   E. Never seen in women

335. This illness is usually characterized by:
   A. Acute onset and relentless deterioration
   B. Uniformly self limiting course
   C. Frequent remissions and exacerbations
   D. Excellent response to penicillin
   E. Excellent response to chloroquine

336. Which one of the following agents is most often useful during
   an acute episode?
   A. Antihistamines   D. Iodo-deoxyuridine
   B. ACTH   E. Tetracycline
   C. BCG vaccination   Ref. 2 - p. 718

CASE (Questions 337-340): A 17 year-old boy had tense, red,
hot, painful swelling of the left knee which was held stiffly in
some flexion. Even slight shaking of the bed caused extreme pain.

337. Your diagnosis is:
   A. Gout   D. Tuberculous arthritis
   B. Traumatic arthritis   E. Joint syphilis
   C. Pyogenic arthritis

338. Which diagnostic procedure is helpful at this time?
   A. X-ray to show destroyed cartilage
   B. Aspiration of joint content for smear and culture
   C. Trial of antibiotic therapy
   D. Blood sedimentation rate
   E. Test for tubercle bacilli in sputum

339. Aspiration of the joint yields thick pus, and history plus physical examination indicate a urethral discharge. Treatment is:
A. Incision, drainage and irrigation plus antibiotic therapy
B. Repeated aspirations
C. Aspiration and antibiotic solution instillation
D. Antibiotic therapy alone
E. Cortisone and X-ray therapy

340. With purulent arthritis, there may be which late result?
A. Joint cartilage destruction and painful motion
B. General septicemia from rupture into soft tissues
C. Fibrous ankylosis with some painful motion
D. Bony ankylosis and painless lack of motion
E. Any of the above   Ref. 4 - p. 1385

CASE (Questions 341-344): An 11 year-old girl is hospitalized because of increasing nervousness and palpitations, after "tranquilizers" provided no relief. Appetite has been good but a weight loss is recorded. School performance has gradually deteriorated and a few "F's" have been reported. The child was sent by the teacher to a guidance counselor and psychiatric help was suggested. On medical examination a wide pulse pressure is found. Skin temperature is increased, excessive perspiration and rapid tendon reflexes were found. The eyes presented a glazed appearance.

341. The most likely diagnosis is:
A. Juvenile thyrotoxicosis   D. Familial dysautonomia
B. Juvenile psychoses   E. Cushing's syndrome
C. Diabetes mellitus

342. Examination should have indicated:
A. Enlargement of thyroid gland   D. Chorea
B. Precocious puberty   E. Splinter hemorrhages
C. Abdominal mass

343. "Eye signs" should have revealed:
A. Nystagmus   D. Lid lag
B. Pin-point vision   E. Uveitis
C. Dilated, fixed pupils

344. Reported complication of therapy with radioactive iodine includes:
A. Thyroid cancer   D. All of the above
B. Leukemia   E. None of the above
C. Permanent hypothyroidism   Ref. 11 - pp. 1313-1315

CASE (Questions 345-348): A 40 year-old male patient with arthritis of several year's duration complains of foul-smelling stools, weight loss and weakness of 3-4 months duration. Physical examination reveals a cachectic patient with low grade fever and prominent lymphadenopathy. Routine laboratory work reveals a moderate anemia, eosinophilia and elevated sedimentation rate. A gluten-free diet fails to result in clinical improvement.

345. A radiological study of the small intestine is likely to resemble that of patients with:
    A. Meckel's diverticulum   D. Regional enteritis
    B. Nontropical sprue   E. Scleroderma
    C. Irritable bowel syndrome

346. Jejunal biopsy is most likely to show:
    A. Normal histology
    B. Periodic acid-Schiff-positive material in macrophages
    C. Increased iron in macrophages
    D. Degeneration of the myenteric plexus
    E. Bacterial overgrowth

347. The patient is most likely to improve after treatment with:
    A. Antibiotics   D. Analgesics
    B. Antihistamines   E. Antacids
    C. Antifolates

348. The diagnosis may also be effectively made by:
    A. Skin biopsy   D. Gastric aspirate
    B. Bone marrow culture   E. Histamine test
    C. Lymph node biopsy   Ref. 2 - p. 1235

CASE (Questions 349-352): A 32 year-old woman had been troubled by progressive dysphagia for several years with necessity to drink water to force food down. There had been no weight loss or loss of appetite but sometimes there was voluminous regurgitation after meals. Recently, there had been several bouts of pneumonia.

349. The most probable diagnosis is:
    A. Esophageal hiatal hernia   D. Esophageal diverticulum
    B. Esophageal achalasia   E. Stricture of the esophagus
    C. Carcinoma of the esophagus

350. Diagnosis is narrowed to achalasia by:
    A. No evidence of gas bubble in stomach above diaphragm
    B. Absence of tumor on esophagoscopy and negative mucosal biopsy
    C. Smooth tapering on esophagoscopy with no inflammation
    D. Absence of barium-filled pouch on esophagogram
    E. All of the above

351. The following statements are correct, except:
    A. Recent pneumonia is due to recumbent overflow
    B. Good appetite and absence of weight loss rule out cancer and stricture
    C. Voluminous regurgitation indicates esophageal dilatation and tortuosity
    D. Esophagoscopy is too dangerous because of the obstruction
    E. Cancer sometimes is associated with achalasia

352. The best treatment in this case is:
    A. Heller esophageal myotomy
    B. Esophagogastrectomy
    C. Repeated blind bouginage
    D. Dilatation by expansile metal dilator
    E. Finger fracture through gastrotomy
                                          Ref. 6 - pp. 1014-1016

CASE (Questions 353-356): A 27 year-old Air Force pilot, seemingly in perfect health, had a routine chest X-ray plate which showed an anterior mediastinal homogeneous density which extended well over both right and left lung shadows. All laboratory and physical findings were normal.

353. The most likely diagnosis is:
    A. Hodgkin's disease   D. Boeck's sarcoid
    B. Thymic cyst   E. Metastatic tumor
    C. Substernal goiter

354. Before thoracotomy, which of the following should be done?
    A. Tomographic films of chest
    B. Bronchoscopy
    C. Lung function studies
    D. GI and GU X-rays looking for a primary tumor
    E. This completely asymptomatic man is ready for thoracotomy now

355. A large cystic thymoma may show which of the following?
    A. Malignancy in its wall
    B. Symptoms and signs of myasthenia gravis
    C. Agammaglobulinemia
    D. All of the above
    E. None of the above

356. Which statement regarding mediastinal tumor is true?
    A. Neural tissue tumors are anteriorly placed
    B. Hodgkin's disease involves the posterior mediastinum
    C. Spring-water and duplication cysts tend to be malignant
    D. Thymoma may be epithelial, lymphoid or teratomatous in origin
    E. Diagnostic trail of X-ray therapy should precede thoracotomy
                                          Ref. 6 - p. 665

For each of the questions or incomplete statements below, one or more of the answers or completions given is correct. Answer according to the following key:

A. If only 1, 2 and 3 are correct
B. If only 1 and 3 are correct
C. If only 2 and 4 are correct
D. If only 4 is correct
E. If all are correct

357. Acute pancreatitis is associated with:
   1. Hyperparathyroidism
   2. Corticosteroids
   3. Pregnancy
   4. Chlorothiazide   Ref. 4 - p. 1103

358. Leiomyosarcoma of the stomach usually causes:
   1. Chronic blood loss
   2. Epigastric pain
   3. Weight loss
   4. Pyloric obstruction   Ref. 6 - p. 1083

359. Solubility of cholesterol in the bile depends on:
   1. Concentration of cholesterol
   2. Concentration of lecithin
   3. Concentration of bile salts
   4. pH of bile   Ref. 4 - p. 1073

360. Contraindications to closed mitral commissurotomy are:
   1. Calcification of the valve
   2. Thrombus in the left atrium
   3. Mitral insufficiency
   4. Atrial fibrillation   Ref. 4 - p. 2055

ANSWER KEY

1. C	51. A	101. D	151. D	201. C
2. C	52. D	102. D	152. A	202. E
3. A	53. C	103. E	153. E	203. B
4. E	54. D	104. A	154. C	204. C
5. C	55. E	105. C	155. A	205. B
6. C	56. E	106. C	156. C	206. A
7. B	57. D	107. E	157. C	207. D
8. C	58. D	108. C	158. D	208. E
9. E	59. B	109. B	159. C	209. A
10. D	60. A	110. E	160. A	210. C
11. B	61. C	111. D	161. B	211. B
12. C	62. E	112. D	162. E	212. E
13. D	63. E	113. D	163. C	213. D
14. E	64. E	114. D	164. C	214. E
15. D	65. B	115. B	165. C	215. A
16. B	66. C	116. C	166. A	216. B
17. D	67. A	117. C	167. C	217. C
18. E	68. C	118. D	168. C	218. D
19. D	69. E	119. D	169. E	219. D
20. B	70. B	120. D	170. A	220. A
21. E	71. D	121. B	171. C	221. E
22. D	72. E	122. C	172. B	222. B
23. B	73. D	123. D	173. C	223. C
24. A	74. A	124. C	174. B	224. C
25. D	75. C	125. C	175. C	225. A
26. E	76. E	126. D	176. E	226. B
27. D	77. B	127. E	177. E	227. D
28. B	78. D	128. D	178. C	228. E
29. D	79. A	129. E	179. B	229. C
30. C	80. E	130. D	180. E	230. E
31. D	81. A	131. D	181. B	231. A
32. B	82. E	132. B	182. B	232. D
33. D	83. A	133. A	183. C	233. B
34. B	84. C	134. C	184. A	234. A
35. E	85. B	135. A	185. A	235. B
36. B	86. A	136. A	186. E	236. D
37. E	87. E	137. C	187. C	237. F
38. C	88. A	138. C	188. B	238. C
39. B	89. B	139. B	189. C	239. B
40. D	90. D	140. E	190. A	240. C
41. A	91. B	141. D	191. D	241. D
42. D	92. D	142. C	192. B	242. A
43. E	93. A	143. E	193. E	243. E
44. C	94. B	144. C	194. B	244. A
45. A	95. E	145. D	195. C	245. B
46. D	96. E	146. B	196. A	246. C
47. C	97. D	147. D	197. C	247. E
48. C	98. E	148. C	198. B	248. D
49. E	99. A	149. B	199. E	249. A
50. B	100. E	150. B	200. A	250. C

ANSWER KEY

251. A	301. A	351. D
252. B	302. D	352. A
253. B	303. E	353. B
254. A	304. A	354. E
255. D	305. A	355. D
256. B	306. A	356. D
257. D	307. C	357. E
258. C	308. B	358. B
259. B	309. C	359. A
260. B	310. B	360. A
261. A	311. D	
262. D	312. D	
263. A	313. D	
264. C	314. C	
265. C	315. B	
266. B	316. D	
267. B	317. C	
268. B	318. B	
269. B	319. A	
270. B	320. B	
271. B	321. B	
272. C	322. C	
273. C	323. E	
274. B	324. D	
275. D	325. C	
276. D	326. C	
277. A	327. C	
278. A	328. B	
279. B	329. B	
280. C	330. B	
281. D	331. C	
282. C	332. D	
283. A	333. E	
284. B	334. C	
285. A	335. C	
286. C	336. B	
287. B	337. C	
288. D	338. B	
289. D	339. A	
290. D	340. E	
291. B	341. A	
292. B	342. A	
293. C	343. D	
294. D	344. D	
295. C	345. B	
296. B	346. B	
297. C	347. A	
298. D	348. C	
299. B	349. B	
300. C	350. E	

REFERENCES

1. Wintrobe, M.M., et al.: Harrison's Principles of Internal Medicine, 7th Ed., McGraw-Hill, 1974.

2. Beeson, P.B. and W. McDermott: Cecil-Loeb, Textbook of Medicine, 14th Ed., Saunders, 1975.

3. Cole, W.H. and R.M. Zollinger: Textbook of Surgery, 9th Ed., Appleton-Century-Crofts.

4. Sabiston, D.C., Jr.: Davis-Christopher Textbook of Surgery, 10th Ed., Saunders, 1972.

5. Rhoads, J.E., et al.: Surgery - Principles and Practice, 4th Ed., Lippincott, 1970.

6. Schwartz, S.I., et al.: Principles of Surgery, 2nd Ed., McGraw-Hill, 1974.

7. Hellman, L.M. and Pritchard, J.A.: Williams Obstetrics, 14th Ed., Appleton-Century-Crofts, 1971.

8. Novak, E.R., et al.: Novak's Textbook of Gynecology, 9th Ed., Williams and Wilkins, 1975.

9. Willson, J.R., et al.: Obstetrics and Gynecology, 4th Ed., revised, Mosby, 1971.

10. Barnett, H.L.: Pediatrics, 15th Ed., Appleton-Century-Crofts, 1972.

11. Vaughan, V.C. and McKay, R.J.: Nelson Textbook of Pediatrics, 10th Ed., Saunders, 1975.